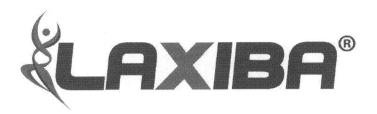

THE FRUCTOSE NAVIGATOR

The Standard for Fructose intolerance

1. Edition

The Nutrition Navigator Books Number Two

M.Sc. J. N. Stratbucker

LAXIBA

Houston

Copyright © 2017 by J. N. Stratbucker

ISBN 978-1-941978-41-2
Library of Congress Control Number 2016905804
Cover design by Mahmood Ali
Interior design by Katharina Maas and Mahmood Ali
Layout by Alexandra Krug
E-Mail of the author: John@Laxiba.com

Laxiba GmbH

Rotweinstrasse 12
53506 Rech
Germany

Victoria Botello
2840 Shadowbriar Drive Apt. 314
Houston, Texas, 77077, USA

For companies and institutions:
Are you interested in bulk orders? Visit us at: *https://laxiba.com*

The data set for the algorithmic ordained statements concerning fructose and sugar alcohols is from the University of Minnesota Nutrition Coordination Center 2014 Food and Nutrient Database. The reason to acquire the database license for this book were its high quality and scope based on international research. Statements regarding fructans and galactans result from six cited international studies. Nevertheless, the contents of the book bear no guarantee. Neither the author, publisher, any cited scientist nor the University of Minnesota is liable for personal injuries or physical or financial damage. Please note that the quantities of critical ingredients in the mentioned products, which are the foundation for the stated portion sizes, are relative and in part based on derivations. The serving sizes in this book are based on approximations of various details. The precise tolerable portion size of any product varies depending on its processing, country-specific composition, degree of maturity and cultivation.

Manufactured in the United States of America

FIRST EDITION

Acknowledgments

Special thanks to M. Thor and the nutritional research team of the University of Minnesota, J. S. Barrett, J. R. Biesiekierski, P. R. Gibson, K. Liels, J. G. Muir, S. J. Shepherd, R. Rose and O. Rosella as well as the rest of the gastroenterology research team of the Monash University, all other cited scientists for their research, B. Hartmann of the Bundesministerium für Ernährung, Landwirtschaft und Verbraucherschutz, G.-W. von Rymon Lipinski of the Goethe University, and H. Zorn of the Justus Liebig University, for copyediting L. Gomes Domingues, F. Lang, C. R. Mundy, L. Popielinski, and M. Vastolo, for their feedback T. Albert, K. Bayer, U. Blendowske, D. Durchdewald, as well as my friends, especially C. Schlick and I. Kloppenburg, and all other contributors who enabled me to write this book in first place.

To my friend K. Warnowizki for always being there for me

Contents

Preface

You just lately learned about your fructose sensitivity? Alternatively, are you well aware of your disease for many years? In each case, this book will help you, as it makes cooking and eating easy with its portion sizes in standard cooking measures as well as in gram and milliliter: scientifically proven and tested by readers like you. You may have tried out expensive medication or radical regimes like the FODMAP diet. Although the latter really works, it is unnecessarily strict. The aim of this book is to bring you more choice while you avoid your symptoms.

The book's information originates from intensive research and interviews with professors. The food tables in this book show you reliable serving sizes for foods concerning fructose intolerance. The design of the tables makes them easy to use. Moreover, they contain several specials. For example, the content of glucose and sorbitol entered the serving size estimations, for results that are more reliable and enable you to eat more of fructose-containing foods by smart combinations.

You do not have to avoid categorically all foods that contain the fructose. It is enough to avoid eating more of them than you can stomach. By having as much choice as possible while preventing your symptoms, you increase your quality of life. How do you know how much your individual sensitivity allows you to eat? Quite simply, this book will tell you. Curious?

Then read on. In the first Chapter, you will learn about the diagnosis, backgrounds and consequences of the disease. Then in Chapter 2, you discover how to implement and keep the diet. You will also find a lot of advice there concerning healthy eating in general, recipes, hints of eating-out, strategies to stay motivated to stress management. Afterward, in Chapter 3 you will find the standard portion sizes for more than 1,000 products. Chapter 4 gives you even more advanced techniques to better adapt to your sensitivity. As I deal with an intolerance for a long time, I know about your need for clarity and practical advice. The focuses of my strategy are quality and suitability for daily use. I wholeheartedly wish you an ongoing success on your way to treat your symptoms and improve your quality of life!

Note: Despite my aim to provide the highest quality, this book should not be the sole basis for any decision you make. Talk about any diet with your doctor before you begin to limit discomfort. You are responsible for your personal health, including how you choose to interpret data and specialists' advice. I cannot guarantee you a recovery. Several causes for your symptoms are possible — to find out more get THE IBS NAVIGATOR.

1

Information

1.1 Why you deserve this book

Congratulations: You take the initiative. By buying this book, you show your will to overcome your discomforts. If you bought this book, you know that a higher well-being is not only good for you but also everyone around you. Turn your back to the symptoms-grumbler. With the proper diet, you will feel healthier and stronger and enjoy more freedom!

Learn all you need to know about your disease, re-evaluate your personal story in that context and learn what you can do to live with it as best as possible. In addition, you find practical advice for a healthier diet in general on page 33 and on page 77 efficient methods to reduce stress, which often worsens your symptoms.

If you bought the book so you could learn to adapt to those in your life suffering from intolerances, you would find out how in Chapter 2.5 and the one following it. Such behavior shows consideration for others that would make anyone glad to be a guest at your table!

That your nutrition affects your happiness is not a secret. It starts with your birth. A full and happy baby makes you happy too. The mother's milk provides the baby with the entire ingredients it needs and tolerates. As an adult, you choose the components of your nutrition yourself. Here it also holds that if you want to be satisfied, you need to eat the food your gut can handle.

Which diagnostic procedure do I have to undergo? Which triggers are possible, which one affects me and how sensitive am I? How much can I eat of foods containing it without hurting myself? Which foods are free of my trigger?

You get the answers for all of the mentioned questions. Explanations of the current scientific results and the most practical food tables for IBS and food intolerances on the market provide you with all you need to take proper action. On top of that, you find the cheat sheets for your wallet that enable you to adapt your diet even when eating out or going to the grocery store. Stop losing valuable energy to abdominal symptoms. Treat them right and start enjoying your life more instead, you deserve it!

1.2 Diagnostic check

Are abdominal pains, bloating, constipation, flatulence or diarrhea your ongoing companion? Without disrespect, we should find a way to get you a better spare time activity. Instead of accepting these discomforts, you should get the appropriate tools to free yourself from them as much as possible in order to spend more of your time enjoying the bright side of life.

The first thing you should do is to find out which of the potential triggers is the one that affects you. Just assuming you have a fructose intolerance is not enough. Going through all diagnostic procedures can take up half a year but will pay off. You will probably be able to get a handle on your symptoms and by using this book, you will also make sure to avoid unnecessary limitations concerning your diet, if you have indeed a sorbitol intolerance—otherwise get *THE IBS, THE LACTOSE* or *THE SORBITOL NAVIGATOR.*

To determine your profile, you should ask your local doctor to send you to an expert, a so-called gastroenterologist. Just the sound of this word might frighten your troublemakers. The specialist then first checks, whether your symptoms have a different cause than an intolerance. The diagnosis will include a **stool analysis**, an **ultrasonic check** and some camera shots inside your stomach to reject other reasons. These tests will allow the specialist to check whether there is an **abnormal bacterial colonization** of the small intestine. This migration may lead to false positives in uncovering an intolerance towards the **main triggers** covered in this book: **fructose, fructans, galactans, lactose,** and **sorbitol**. The next test looks for **celiac disease**, sensitivity towards gluten, which is an ingredient in grains. In people who have an untreated celiac disease, the tolerance test for the cube sorbitol is often positive, even if they can stomach it if they avoid gluten-containing foods. Following this, you should take a genetic test regarding **hereditary fructose** intolerance. Hereditary fructose intolerance is rare, but it is serious: the fructose test itself can be lethal to those with this disease. If you are affected, you have to abstain from fructose. Use the big smileys in the fructose tables to find fructose free foods.

You ruled out other potential causes, and the brats are probably trembling. Great, as now they are in for: what follows are checks regarding three of the mentioned main triggers. For the so-called breath test, you will take a high dose containing fructose, lactose or sorbitol on different days. If one of these passes through to your large intestine, due to suboptimal absorption by your body, gasses emerge. The doctors measure them to find out if you have an intolerance. When the amount of gas reaches a certain level, the diagnosis is an intolerance toward the respective trigger and have to adapt your diet accordingly. The threshold for a positive diagnosis for a fructose dilution (typically containing 25–50g) is usually 20ppm (parts per million, a concentration measure). This threshold also applies for lactose and sorbitol. The recommended breath test, however, is not available everywhere. In Chapter 2.2.1 you will learn about a substitute test, in case you have no access to the breath test.

Has the breath or substitute test shown that your body has enough capacity to handle even extreme amounts of a trigger? If so, you do not need to take any further attention to the trigger; its consumption will not cause you any harm—ignore the trigger: there is no point in taking unnecessary diets. If however the test shows that you have for example an intolerance towards fructose, you know which of the triggers you have to render harmless by limiting your consumption of foods in which it is present.

In general, do not accept a diagnosis without a test. If none of the tests comes to a conclusive result, you have an irritable bowel syndrome that is at least—for now—undefined. Irritable bowel just means that your gut reacts sensitively to various types of irritations such as gasses inside it—more on that in Chapter 1.4. The bowel is the final segment of your alimentary canal and the section where your symptoms come to show. Irritable bowel symptoms can be defined—if you have one of the before mentioned intolerances or undefined. If it is undefined, either, you did not take a test or it showed that you do not have an intolerance to one of the mentioned triggers. Note here that no breath-test is available for fructans and galactans as of now, and you need my *IBS* book to test it. In both cases, the symptoms are similar, because readily fermentable carbohydrates, a group that all triggers belong to, of some sort trigger the symptoms. Incidentally, for up to 90% of patients with IBS, an intolerance to one or more of the three breath-test-triggers mentioned above causes the symptoms.

If you suffer from irritable bowel symptoms, you are not alone: 20% of Americans have an intolerance, i.e., their enzyme worker team is too small for one or more of the three triggers that one tests with a breath test. Worldwide, 10–15% of all people suffer from undefined abdominal discomfort. About 20–30% of Europeans in general, 9% of the Dutch, 22% of the English, 25% of the Japanese and 44% of West Africans are affected. Concerning children, they should only take a diet under medical supervision. By the way, a lactose intolerance can only evolve at an age above five years. All younger children can stomach lactose.

It is also possible that a doctor finds that you are intolerant according to a breath test, but you do not feel symptoms. In such a case you may still want to keep the respective diet if you suffer from depressive moods, see Chapter 1.3.3.

Summary

If you regularly suffer from abdominal discomfort, visit a specialist, a gastroenterologist. You may assume you have a fructose intolerance but only a specialist can rule out more severe diseases. Checks can take up to half a year. Many others share your fate; about 20% of Americans are affected. You are holding in your hands the key to fighting the symptoms!

1.3   Presentation of the triggers

We depict fructose as cubes. Why? Just imagine having a big cube in your stomach. Not a good feeling. On the other hand, a cube can have a positive effect, too. Think of a sugar cube that provides a lot of energy. Likewise, fructose, being sugar related carbohydrate, provides you with energy, if your stomach makes use for it in that way.

1.3.1   How symptoms emerge

If you have an intolerance against fructose, your body only provides a few workers making sure your body uses the cube for energy. Few workers mean that if you eat too much of foods that contain fructose cubes, many remain un-used by your body and arrive at your large intestine. Now, two processes are responsible for the symptoms: osmosis and fermentation. To understand osmosis, let us imagine two equal fish bowls connected by an underwater tube.

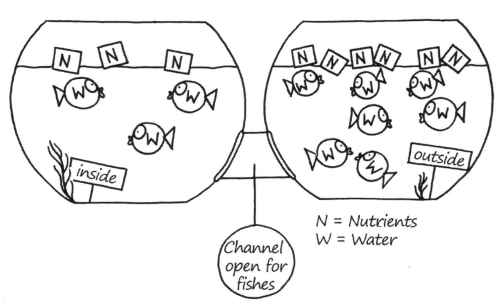

The glass on the left represents the inside of the bowel and the one on the right for the outside of it. The fishes represent water (W), and their food are either nutrient (N) or fructose cubes that arrive at the inside of the bowel (F). The channel enables fishes to switch between the bowls. Thus, they always swim to the glass that contains more food. Usually, this would be the outside of the intestine. Thereby, the body detracts the water from the foods—which is a good.

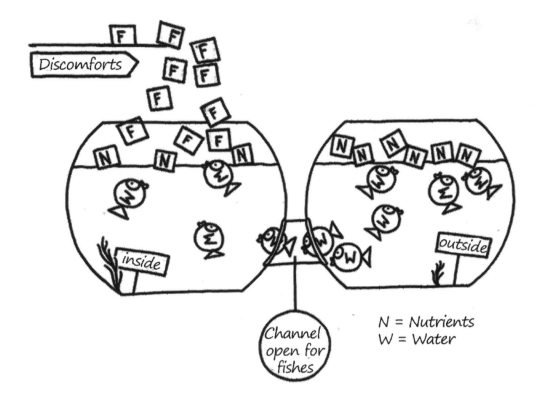

However, if you eat more of foods containing fructose than your enzyme workers can handle, fructose cubes arrive at the inside of the bowel. Hence, suddenly there is more food in the left fish bowl.

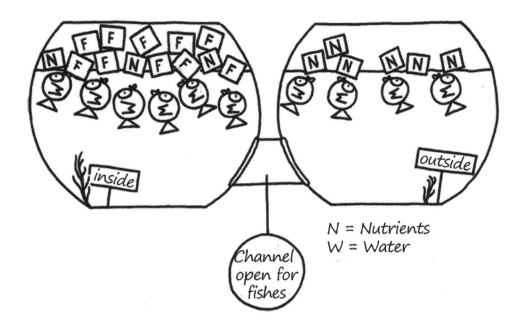

N = Nutrients
W = Water

As the intestinal wall, here represented by the channel, is only partially permeable, the fishes can swim through it, unlike the food. Therefore, some fishes now switch sides and scrimmage on the left. Their movement to the left means that with the cubes water arrives inside the intestine and you suffer from diarrhea.

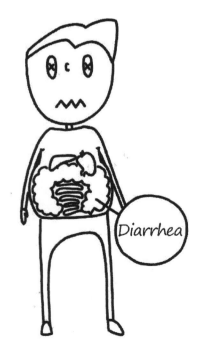

Now you know about osmosis. What causes fermentation?
As you know, you have bacteria inside your bowel, which is normal and that way for any healthy person. The issue is that these bacteria love sweets. Hence, if a fructose cube arrives at the large intestine, they do not falter and immediately consume it to help themselves to some energy.

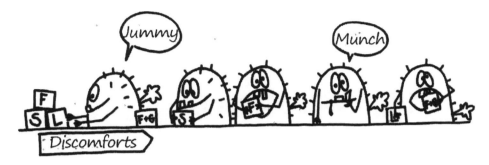

Unfortunately, though, the bacteria are less efficient at consuming fructose cubes than our body is. When bacteria use fructose cubes, gas emerges.

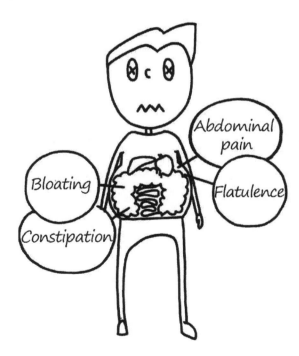

The gas either leaves as bloating or amounts and causes an uncomfortable flatulence. If the pressure increases in some regions of the intestines, this can cause deposits—constipation. If the gas enters the small intestine, it causes, even more, turmoil: it hinders some of thebody's cube workers from doing their job. That is because the workers mainly sit on the gut wall and the gas reduces its contact to the stool. However, what about the treatment with a diet? In general, it is important for your health to have a diverse diet. The FODMAP approach, which you may have heard of, aims at reducing the fermentation and osmosis by lowering the consumption of all potential triggers at once. With the fructose standard treatment of this book, you take a more precise aim to give you more freedom concerning your food choice. With it, you only avoid fructose and the equivalent amount of sorbitol as explained in the following. First, you should get to know it, though.

1.3.2   Fructose characteristics

Fruit naturally contains fructose, and that is why another name for it is fruit sugar. Some fruits, like Rhubarb, are free from it, though. Nowadays, fructose is the cause of the sweet taste of many foods. It enters the ingredients as honey, gelling sugars, and corn syrup. In the absence of an intolerance, humans can smoothly break down fructose. Luckily, even in case you do have a fructose intolerance you can consume some of it and to your benefit, foods that contain glucose and enhance your tolerance as shown below.

   The way you mainly take in fructose depends on your nutritional habits. In the USA, about two-thirds are taken in as soft drinks, enriched convenience foods, and about one-third as fruit. In Finland, the relations are the other way around. For 39% of those affected by unexplained regular abdominal discomfort, symptoms arise after the consumption of 15g fructose; for 70%, they appear after a dose of 30g. People around the globe consume between 11 and 54g per day, or 4-18g per meal. The following illustrations show you, what happens in the case of a fructose intolerance.

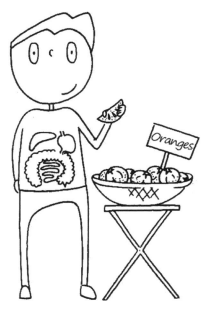

Man <u>with</u> fructose intolerance

Oranges naturally contain fructose: John has a fructose intolerance and therefore only has a piece of it at breakfast. He knows that he only has a few conveyor belt worker that make sure his body assimilates fructose.

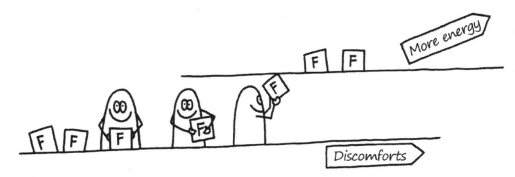

With the amount contained in one piece, his workers can cope—as long as he avoids eating any more products that contain fructose. Thus, his body assimilates the fructose he ate (F), turns it into energy and abdominal discomforts are absent.

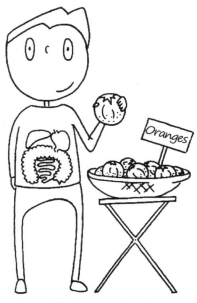

Man <u>with</u> fructose intolerance

However, now John forgets that his team is quite an observable one and eats a whole orange at once. Thus, he makes it sweat a lot.

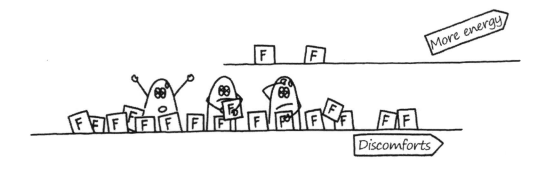

His workers are unable to cope with the sudden fructose load and leave most of it on the belt. This redundant fructose arrives at the large intestine, and there it triggers symptoms.

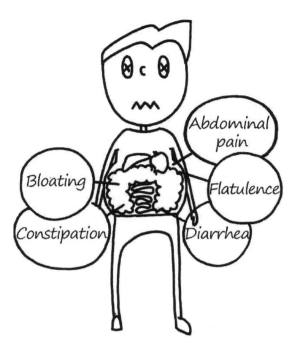

A few hours after the consumption the following symptoms can occur: abdominal pain, bloating, diarrhea and flatulence.

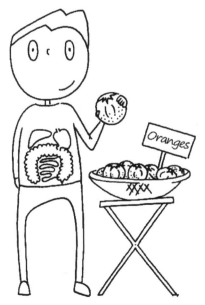

Man *without* fructose intolerance

When Chris, who does not have a fructose intolerance, eats a whole orange, it is a different ball game.

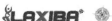

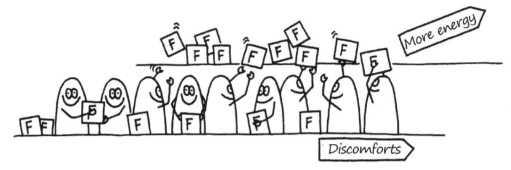

As he has many more fructose employees on the conveyor belt, these handle the load with ease.

Hereditary fructose intolerance

If you suffer from the rare and unfortunately not yet curable hereditary fructose intolerance, consuming fructose can be lethal. Please seek your doctor's advice. You can use the food table in this book to determine foods that are free of fructose. Only eat those with a big smile in the fructose column.

Folic acid deficiency

A folic acid deficiency increases the risk of cardiovascular disease. A fructose intolerance often negatively affects folic acid absorption. Hence, it would be sensible to take suitable supplements. Otherwise, folic acid is contained in Kellogg's® Corn Flakes (323µg/100g), some protein powders (280µg/100g) and short-grain rice (225µg/100g), for example. The recommended daily dose is 300µg for men, 250µg for most women and 400µg for expectant mothers.

Influence of glucose

Glucose does the job for the fructose workers. As soon as glucose meets fructose in effect, they act as if they combined to form table sugar. As you can tolerate much more table sugar than fructose, you can benefit from this effect. To do that, you have to mix food that contains fructose with food containing an equal amount of glucose either in advance or in your mouth.

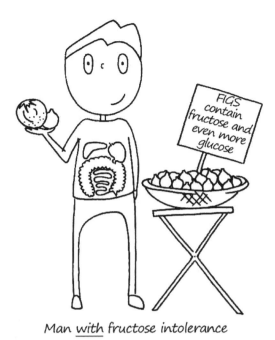

Man <u>with</u> fructose intolerance

As John still loves eating oranges, he now eats it together with a fig, which contains a lot of glucose.

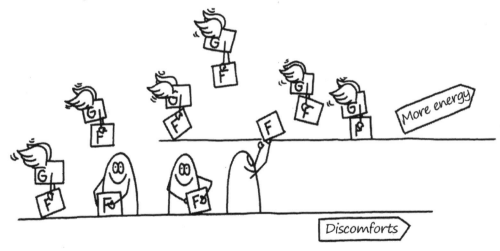

The glucose does it jobs and John's body quickly assimilates the glucose-fructose couple to energy. Despite the fructose load of a whole orange, his team now has a walkover.

Foods that have an abundance of glucose

The following foods are free of other triggers like lactose, sorbitol, and contain a lot of glucose. When consumed with food that is limited by fructose, you can increase the limit by the factors in the following table. If you are interested, just test it out for yourself. You find your multiplier in one of the last four columns of the next table.

Foods	Portion weight	Amount multiplier per portion
Avocado (Florida)	37.5 g	2.25
Fresh figs	50 g	2.0
Maple syrup	30 g	1.5
Mozzarella	28g	1.25
Sweet corn	82g	3.25
Thin slice of pineapple	56.3g	2.25

You can also purchase pure glucose as a powder online though you should avoid a high sugar consumption due to potential health implications (see Chapter 2.1.4).

Influence of sorbitol

Sorbitol and fructose mostly share the same workers. However, if you consume foods that contain sorbitol together with some that contain fructose, the workers always handle sorbitol first. As fewer workers are thus handling the fructose, more remains on the discomforts belt—ends up in the large intestine. For that reason, I accounted for the sorbitol content when estimating the fructose portion sizes you find in the food tables in Chapter 3. The following illustration shows you the interaction of fructose and sorbitol:

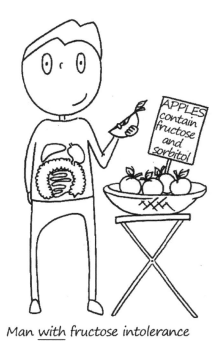

Man <u>with</u> fructose intolerance

Now John eats a piece of apple despite his fructose intolerance…

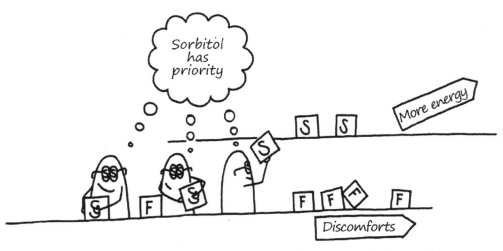

… as an apple contains sorbitol in addition to fructose, and the workers love to handle it most, fructose is left on the belt, and John has symptoms despite eating only a piece.

The impact of sorbitol

Those that do not have a fructose intolerance have enough workers to cope with both fructose and sorbitol. At the utmost, the sorbitol that you consume at a meal can hinder the absorption of the equal amount of fructose by your body. An apple contains 0.56g of sorbitol at most and about 4g of fructose. Thereby the sorbitol contained in an apple can block the handling of 0.56g of fructose at most. Thereby, sorbitol is only an issue for you, as long as you solely suffer from a fructose intolerance, if you consume it together with fructose. If you would add the respective amount of glucose to a glass of apple juice, you could even spare yourself of fructose symptoms entirely as the glucose acts as if it connects to the fructose to form table sugar and sorbitol does not affect this. Therefore, in the case of a sole fructose intolerance, sorbitol is a mere symptoms promoter. In the fructose tables in Chapter 3, the amount of sorbitol that blocks fructose entered the tolerable serving size algorithm according to the example above.

Foods that contain sorbitol

Various fruits and vegetables contain sorbitol. In extreme amounts, you can find it in many products that are sugar-free or for diabetics. Often sorbitol only shows up as the numeric code 420. You should adjust to it in case you are fructose or sorbitol intolerant. Important: If you only have a fructose but not a sorbitol intolerance, it is enough if you eat according to the fructose portions in Chapter 3 as sorbitol has already been accounted for here.

Your personal sensitivity

The amount of fructose that you should limit yourself to per meal is different from person to person. For that reason, you can try whether you can, for example, stomach twice the amount in this book's tables. The standard amount you can tolerate in the case of fructose intolerance is 0.5g of fructose that is unmatched by glucose.

Enzyme capsules

Xylose isomerase is available on the market. The author is aware of only one study that aimed to prove its efficiency, and it showed symptoms improving by about 41%. Whether this justifies the current high sales price, remains for you to decide.

1.3.3 Consequences of a fructose intolerance

Physical effects

You are already familiar with the immediate effects of an untreated fructose intolerance: abdominal pain, bloating, diarrhea and flatulence. These alone are certainly enough to have you take action. However, indirectly they can also lead to lower lust, reduced social contacts, lower empathy and less vitality in general. Hence, not handling your intolerance lowers your quality of life. It is not so surprising that this also affects your days off work. A study, done in the USA and the Netherlands, shows that on average people with an untreated intolerance take about twice as many sick leaves from school or work than do their peers. Luckily, you can do something about that. You can recapture your wellbeing by learning how to adapt your diet to your capacity to absorb fructose. Ideally, you only limit your nutrition as far as is necessary—a certain amount of fructose is usually even tolerable if you are intolerant towards fructose. My aim is to make this as easy as possible for you.

Depression

Scientists have found that there is a causal relation between having an untreated intolerance and increased depression scores. The reason for this is a reduced prevalence of a neurotransmitter, serotonin, in case fructose arrives at the large intestine. Serotonin elevates one's mood. The body produces it from tryptophan, which it derives from food. Presumably, at least, fructose that passes the small intestine—remains on the belt—merges with tryptophan to form a non-absorbable substance. This reaction reduces the amount of available tryptophan and causes the body to produce less serotonin. Hence, fructose that arrives at the large intestine hinders the body's ability to let positive feelings emerge. In an experiment in which patients lowered their fructose consumption, depression scores normalized for most participants. Keeping the consumption limits that apply to you when choosing your portion sizes can improve your mood (your serotonin metabolism) because fewer fructose arrives at the large intestine. Extra discipline is required to maintain the portion thresholds in cases of depression, however, as a lack of high spirits (tryptophan) can foster the hunger for sweets. Now, candies often contain fructose. If an intolerance is present, the intake of fructose containing sweets further lowers one's mood, creating a vicious circle. You can find out how much you can eat for many foods in the lists in Chapter 3. Even if you are not depressed, please remember that in the presence of a dysfunctional metabolism, depression can result from consuming too much of foods that contain problematic ingredients. Affected people should always seek help rather than trying to counter these effects through sheer willpower and bear in mind that they can and should do something about ongoing feelings of sadness, little personal power, and low energy.

 ## Summary

Fructose is a carbohydrate that bacteria ferment if it reaches the large intestine. In that case, it causes various abdominal symptoms. Many foods contain fructose. In case of a fructose intolerance, you have too few enzyme workers making sure your body uses fructose to gain energy before it can reach the large intestine. You treat your symptoms by limiting your consumption of fructose to the capacity of your enzyme workers. To do so, you eat according to the tables in the third Chapter showing you the tolerated amount per meal. The algorithm I invented for that considers the amount of sorbitol for the first time. Thereby, the portion sizes are more reliable. Moreover, I also show you foods that contain glucose. If you consume these with fructose containing foods, you can enhance the amount you tolerate. Hence, I help you with avoiding your symptoms, and enjoying as much freedom as is possible concerning your choice of foods.

1.4   Background of an irritable bowel

Suffering from a fructose intolerance is like having a sensitive colon. Like a notorious diva, the intestine shows a lack of robustness and an over-sensitivity. It will not allow tampering with, reacts disappointed and offended when ignored by someone that offers her unfitting food. In the case of stress, she pipes up even more vehemently. Many people are carrying such a diva around with them, which repeatedly makes her demands known.

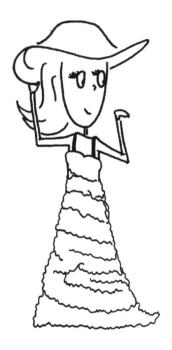

By the way, the exact causes of the diva's show up are unknown. In some cases, infections and emotions play a role. It seems like fortune decided who has a fructose intolerance and who does not. In any case, it has nothing to do with the character. Having a diva-tummy not at all means having a diva-like congeniality.

1.5   Abdominal discomfort in kids

In general, abdominal discomforts of your child can have a variety of reasons. A lactose intolerance will not occur before the age of five. Other potential triggers of abdominal pain, bloating and diarrhea in children are fructose and sorbitol: Children ages 14 to 58 months drank 250 ml of apple juice in a study. Afterward, all children who suffered from chronic diarrhea, as well as 65.5% of the healthy children, tested positive for malabsorption-symptoms. Avoiding apple juice led to recovery for **all** of the children. This result corresponds with other research that shows that many children suffer from diarrhea and abdominal pain if they drink too much fruit juice. Liquids that contain high levels of sorbitol are often the trigger. You should give your child a maximum of 10 ml juice per kilogram of body weight. Moreover, you should avoid giving them fruit juices that contain sorbitol or high amounts of free fructose, like apple or peach juice.

2

STRATEGY

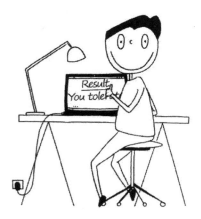

2.1   A gut's change management

No employee likes to stay at a company that always overstrains him. Equally unsatisfactory is to work at a place where one gets the feeling that one does not contribute at all. The typical consequences of both extremes: lack of motivation, an increase in the number of sick leaves up to an incapacity to work at the place anymore. What does that have to do with you? Quite simply: what goes in the professional environment, applies to your bowel as well. Hence, you should strive to work with your enzymes (conveyor-belt workers) in a team instead of over- or under-straining them. Show your leadership qualities and make your staff your motivated allies instead of waiting for them to come to you with their complaints!

How you can get that done, you will find out in this book. Did you ever want to rely on a master plan? If that is so, you will like what follows. According to the following plan, you will first determine the status quo of your symptoms. The next step is to keep a fructose diet for three weeks. At the end you determine, whether your symptoms have improved. If so, you can find out whether you can stomach more than the standard amounts—better adapt to the capacity of your workers. If your symptoms did not improve to your satisfaction, work on your stress level according to Chapter 2.8 or get THE IBS NAVIGATOR to search for alternative triggers.

2.1.1 Signpost

Status-quo-check:	Introduction diet:	Efficiency check:	Adaption:
Note down your symptoms for four days **before** the diet	Keep the the fructose diet according to the food tables in Chapter 3.	Note down your symptoms on the last four days of your introductory diet to determine if the diet worked. If not, check alternative causes.	Sensitivity check to find out if you can tolerate more than the standard serving sizes.

2.1.2　Roadmap

Step	Action	Target
Duty 1	**Status-quo-check** Fill out the symptom test sheet Duration: 4 days	Determining your status quo: Which symptoms do you have, and how severe are they?
Optional 2	**Breath tests at a specialist** Duration: 4 days	As you bought this book, you have either already taken it or done the substitute test in *THE IBS NAVIGATOR*. Otherwise, you can take the introductory diet to find out if the fructose diet works for you but it is more advisable to check for alternative triggers as well and for that, you need the book or a breath test.
Duty 3	**Introductory diet and efficiency check with symptom test sheet** Symptom tracking during the last four days of the diet. Duration of the diet: three weeks	You keep the fructose diet with the Chapter 3 tables and fill out the symptom test sheet. Did the diet lower your symptoms satisfactory? **Yes)** Continue with step four. **No)** Work on the stress management chapter. Another option is to check alternative triggers and diseases with *THE IBS NAVIGATOR*.
Optional 4	**Sensitivity-level-test** Duration: ~½ month	Enabling you a diet that is as varied as possible while reducing your symptoms is possible by determining your sensitivity level, see Chapter 4.

The goal of the overall strategy is to determine how much you tolerate without causing "the diva" to protest. The first step towards that goal it to determine the status quo, the severity of your symptoms, before changing your diet. The reason for this is that this is the only way to check, whether the diet has an effect. To do so, note down your discomforts in a copy of the following symptom test sheet. **Make sure to keep your symptom test sheets in a folder.** The days at which you note down your symptoms should be average to you. Neither a day on which you sickly vegetated in your bed nor one on which you celebrated the stag party of your best friend or had to master a difficult test count. If you are uncertain about whether it was an average day, cross it out. **Important: This also holds true for all of the subsequent tests. If you are in doubt as to whether the day was "normal," i.e. no circumstances distorted the symptoms, repeat the test to get a more reliable result.** On the days where you track your symptoms, always carry a copy of the symptom test sheet with you. Ideally, you should fill it out right after your main meals, e.g., at 7 am, 1 pm and 7 pm. After the four days of your status quo check, you should also be able to classify the type of stool you usually have. Depending on whether you have constipation, diarrhea or a mix of both, you are an IBS-C, IBS-D or IBS-M type. If you have neither constipation nor diarrhea, your IBS type is unclassified. Take that information with you when you visit the doctor. After tracking your symptoms for four days, follow the introductory diet. That means you keep a diet according to the tables in Chapter 3. In the last week, you then fill out the symptom test sheet to determine the diet's effectiveness. If keeping the diet leads to an improvement of your well-being that you are satisfied with, you should stick to it. You can read how to assess the test sheets more professionally than just laying the one before next to the one after the diet in Chapter 4.3. You can use the efficiency-check-symptom-sheet later as a reference for the sensitivity-level-test, if you decide to take it—it is also included in the advanced techniques-Chapter 4. With the latter, you can adjust to your enzyme worker's capacities to handle fructose.

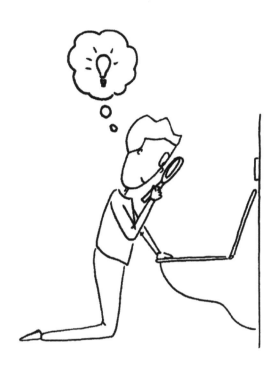

Stool types after Bristol

	Separate hard lumps, like nuts (hard to pass)	**Type** A: Constipation **Value** 4
	Sausage-shaped but lumpy	**Type** B: Constipation Value 2
	Like a sausage but with cracks on the surface	**Type** C: normal **Value** 1
	Like a sausage or snake, smooth and soft	**Type** D: normal **Value** 1
	Soft blobs with clear-cut edges	**Type** E: Diarrhea **Value** 2
	Fluffy pieces with ragged edges, a mushy stool	**Type** F: Diarrhea **Value** 4
	Watery, no solid pieces; **entirely liquid**	**Type** G: Diarrhea **Value** 5

(Based on Lewis & Heaton, 1997; Thompson, 2006)

Types 3 and 4 are the norm. The farther away your type is from these two, the worse your ailments.

2.1.3 Symptom test sheet

Note down your stool type in the morning 🐓, afternoon ☀, and evening ☾ and your stool value from 1 to 5 (see page 28) as well as the number of times you visited the toilet to estimate the stool grade by multiplying the numbers. Also, evaluate bloating and pain from 1 to 5 according to the following scale:

1 No discomfort, like someone without symptoms
2 Hardly any discomfort relative to someone without symptoms
3 Medium discomfort relative to someone without symptoms
4 Severe discomfort relative to someone without symptoms
5 Very severe discomfort relative to someone without symptoms

Test:_____ **End date:**_____

For each test, you need copies of this page!

		Type/ Value	Defecation count	Stool grade	+	Bloating grade	+	Pain grade	= B	
Day 1 prior	🐓		x	=						**TEST DAY**
	☀		x	=(+)		+		+		
	☾		x	=(+)		+		+		
		The day's sum	**A =**	=		=				
Day 2 prior	🐓		x	=						**Day 1 after**
	☀		x	=(+)		+		+		
	☾		x	=(+)		+		+		
		The day's sum	**A =**	=		=				
Day 3 prior	🐓		x	=						**Day 2 after**
	☀		x	=(+)		+		+		
	☾		x	=(+)		+		+		
		The day's sum	**A =**	=		=				
Day 4 prior)	🐓		x	=						**Day 3 after**
	☀		x	=(+)		+		+		
	☾		x	=(+)		+		+		
		The day's sum	**A =**	=		=				

Example: The four status quo (1.)/Level (2.) check days

Note down your stool type in the morning 🐓, afternoon ☀, and evening ☾ and your stool value from 1 to 5 (see page 28) as well as the number of times you visited the toilet to estimate the stool grade by multiplying the numbers. Also, evaluate bloating and pain from 1 to 5 according to the following scale:

1   No discomfort, like someone without symptoms
2   Hardly any discomfort relative to someone without symptoms
3   Medium discomfort relative to someone without symptoms
4   Severe discomfort relative to someone without symptoms
5   Very severe discomfort relative to someone without symptoms

Test:_____   End date:_____

For each test, you need copies of this page!

		Type/ Value	Defecation count		Stool grade	Bloating grade	Pain grade	
Day 1 prior	🐓	E 2	x 2	=	4	2	2	**TEST DAY**
	☀	F 4	x 2	=(+)	8	+ 2	+ 3	
	☾	E 2	x 2	=(+)	4	+ 3	+ 2	
			The day's sum	=	16	= 7	= 7	
Day 2 prior	🐓	F 4	x 2	=	8	2	3	**Day 1 after**
	☀	E 2	x 1	=(+)	2	+ 3	+ 4	
	☾	F 4	x 1	=(+)	4	+ 2	+ 2	
			The day's sum	=	14	= 7	= 9	
Day 3 prior	🐓	E 2	x 1	=	2	2	3	**Day 2 after**
	☀	F 4	x 2	=(+)	8	+ 2	+ 4	
	☾	E 2	x 1	=(+)	2	+ 3	+ 5	
			The day's sum	=	12	= 7	= 12	
Day 4 prior)	🐓	F 4	x 1	=	4	2	2	**Day 3 after**
	☀	E 2	x 1	=(+)	2	+ 2	+ 2	
	☾	F 4	x 2	=(+)	8	+ 3	+ 3	
			The day's sum	=	14	= 7	= 7	

Example: The four efficiency check days

Note down your stool type in the morning 🐓, afternoon ☀, and evening ☾ and your stool value from 1 to 5 (see page 28) as well as the number of times you visited the toilet to estimate the stool grade by multiplying the numbers. Also, evaluate bloating and pain from 1 to 5 according to the following scale:

1 No discomfort, like someone without symptoms
2 Hardly any discomfort relative to someone without symptoms
3 Medium discomfort relative to someone without symptoms
4 Severe discomfort relative to someone without symptoms
5 Very severe discomfort relative to someone without symptoms

Test:_____ **End date:**_____

For each test, you need copies of this page!

		Type/ Value	Defecation count	Stool grade	Bloating grade	Pain grade	
Day 1 prior	🐓	-	x 0	= 0	1	1	**TEST DAY**
	☀	E 2	x 1	=(+) 2	+ 1	+ 1	
	☾	D 1	x 1	=(+) 1	+ 1	+ 1	
		The day's sum		= 3	= 3	= 3	
Day 2 prior	🐓	D 1	x 1	= 1	1	1	**Day 1 after**
	☀	-	x 0	=(+) 0	+ 1	+ 1	
	☾	D 1	x 1	=(+) 1	+ 1	+ 1	
		The day's sum		= 2	= 3	= 3	
Day 3 prior	🐓	D 1	x 1	= 1	1	1	**Day 2 after**
	☀	-	x 0	=(+) 0	+ 2	+ 2	
	☾	E 2	x 1	=(+) 2	+ 1	+ 1	
		The day's sum		= 3	= 4	= 4	
Day 4 prior)	🐓	-	x 0	= 0	1	1	**Day 3 after**
	☀	D 1	x 1	=(+) 1	+ 1	+ 1	
	☾	D 1	x 1	=(+) 1	+ 1	+ 1	
		The day's sum		= 2	= 3	= 3	

2.1.4   Keeping your balance

Now, you know if the diet provides you benefits and maybe even, how sensitive you are. Still, aside from avoiding the consumption of too much of your trigger, you should also learn some generally advisable nutrition principles.

1	Eat a rich variety of foods, i.e., something different each day and with lots of natural ingredients. Eat with a relaxed posture.	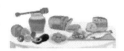
2	Take care of your supply of fiber, e.g., by eating potatoes, flax seeds, lentils, nuts.	
3	Ingest five portions of vegetables (ideally dark green, red or orange) and fruit.	5/day
4	Have some reduced-fat milk products like reduced-fat milk, yogurt or cheese every day.	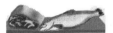
5	One or two times a week, eat fish and eggs, as well as 300–600g of low-fat meat, ideally poultry.	
6	Use vegetable oils if possible, like canola oil, and fats.	
7	Reduce your consumption of salt and sugar.	
8	Drink at least 1.5 liters of non-alcoholic drinks per day. Best are unsweetened beverages and water. Drink alcohol moderately or avoid it entirely.	
9	Preferably, cook fresh and at lower temperatures to reduce nutrient leaching.	
+	Stay fit: exercise regularly.	

◈ Summary

As part of the strategy, you first note down your symptoms before doing anything. Then you start the introductory diet. For it, you reduce the consumption of fructose. The aim is to check whether the diet lowers your symptoms after all. So, fill out the symptom-test-sheet before starting the diet. Then follow the diet according to the tables in Chapter 3 for three weeks and fill out the test-sheet once more for the last four days. If you are feeling better now, you can also determine your precise sensitivity level; see Chapter 4. If you still have symptoms, follow steps two and three as described on the next page.

Make sure you keep a balanced diet:
    Drink least 1.5 liters of water per day and exercise regularly. Also, ensure to eat a variety of foods, to supply your body with the vitamins that are important for your health. To achieve that, regularly eat fruits and vegetables.

2.2 Your individual strategy

This Chapter describes how to proceed accurately with the introduction of diet and the sensitivity level test. During the introductory diet you keep the portions stated in the tables in Chapter 3. Please note here that the tolerated portions refer to one meal—expecting three meals at intervals of about six hours per day. Follow these steps to find out if the diet has an effect:

First, you take the introductory diet for fructose. Four days before starting the diet as well as on the last four days of the third week, you fill out the symptom test sheet on page 29. With it, you can determine the diet's success, see chapter 4.3. The diet is efficient; however, if after three weeks of keeping it, you should not find any improvement, find out whether you unwillingly consumed too much fructose. One way to do so is to keep a nutrition diary and check it with a specialist or nutrition consultant. If you ruled out an accidental intake of the fructose and are unhappy with the improvement of your well-being, make sure to work on your stress management see Chapter 2.8. Aside from that, you can use *THE IBS NAVIGATOR* to test for a fructans and galactans sensitivity and perform alternative strategies.

The test procedure in three levels of escalation

Subsequently, you find an example of the test process:
1) Reduce your fructose consumption according to the tables in Chapter 3 for three weeks. Fill out the symptom test sheet for four days before the diet as well as on the last four days. In the third week, if your discomforts improved satisfactory, keep the fructose diet. If you like, you can adjust your sensitivity level further (see Chapter 4). If you remain dissatisfied, act according to step 2).
2) Improve your stress management according to Chapter 2.8.
3) Get *THE IBS NAVIGATOR* and repeat the introduction with fructans and galactans as well. Did your symptoms improve further? If so, keep this diet. In case you are still searching for an improvement, check the alternative strategies chapter in that book.

2.2.1 Substitute test

You want to check, whether you can stomach fructose but your expert is unable to offer you a breath test? For this case, I have developed the substitute test. As you determine the result based on your symptoms, it is necessary to rule out the influence of alternative triggers. Thus, you need *THE IBS NAVIGATOR* to do the test. In it, you will find the extensive explanation and the instruction to perform the substitute test.

2.2.2 It depends on the total load

You feel discomfort as soon as too much of fructose arrives at your small intestine for your enzyme workers to handle. The more fructose, the worse your symptoms are. In the food tables in the third part of the book, you will find the portion sizes that fit your level. What do you do if you want to combine different foods, e.g., as you prepare to cook a recipe, if you tolerate a limited amount of some of them? If you used the maximum amount of fructose on the apple pie, do you have to deny yourself the raspberrys with vanilla sauce? Nonessential: reduce the consumption for one or several of the affected foods far enough to not surpass the amount thresholds in sum. Makes sense? Not yet? Here is another example: you want to eat pineapple as a snack (the tolerable amount is ¾ of a portion of 140g) together with orange (your acceptable portion size for it is 2¼ of a portions of 140g). Hence, both foods contain fructose. In order not to surpass your tolerance threshold, restrict yourself to ¼ of a portion of pineapple and one portion of orange. Thus, the total amount of fructose you consume at the meal is below your threshold. If the reduced amounts are too small for you, you may want to combine the two with foods like figs that contain more glucose than fructose and increase the amount of fructose you tolerate, if you consume them at the same time. You can recognize them by the smiley with a plus in the food tables. In addition, you can use fructose free alternatives, like rhuarb. In Chapter 3.7.1, you can find various fruits.

2.3   Prevalence of the intolerances

According to an extensive current study in Switzerland, 27% of people with abdominal discomfort suffer from a fructose intolerance, 17% from a lactose intolerance and a further 33% from both. However, the fructose dose of 35g that the study used is high for European conditions, if a Finnish study from 1987 still applies to contemporary diets, and low for American conditions, wherein the average daily amount consumed is 54g. Hence, there is no fixed reference around the world. Another research study using 25g fructose as its base level suggests only a 49% average prevalence of fructose intolerance. An analysis of several studies shows that independent from the investigations mentioned above, 58% of those with irritable bowel symptoms have a sorbitol intolerance. There are no research results concerning the prevalence of a fructans and galactans intolerance known to me at this point.

Are you surprised about the low level of lactose intolerance? Well, you have to account for the fact that it is lowest for Caucasians as they adapted to tolerate milk to cope better with less sunshine in a day. Still, I was amazed that lactose intolerance is not the common type of intolerances according to the studies I read. If you stroll through supermarkets, however, you will hardly find a shelf that holds products for people with sorbitol or fructose intolerance. Instead, the markets have adjusted solely on lactose intolerance—also concerning the labeling. From this perspective, it is better to be lactose intolerant. Those suffering from fructose intolerance have to know sorbitol (and maybe all the difficult names of the other sugar alcohols) as well as fructose due to interaction effects.

2.4   General diet hints

2.4.1   Good reasons for your persistence

I magine that one of your best friends goes on a two-week vacation leaving his beloved Labrador retriever, *Bailey*, in your care, along with some instructions about the dog's health needs as it has an intolerance towards an ingredient in some dog foods. You run out of dog food after the first week, just as you sat down on the couch to relax—not planning to leave the house again for today. Now you remember that you still have a can of the food you give to the square like dog of your auntie in the basement. If you give *Bailey* some of that, you save an hour drive to the store and back as well as going outside where it started to rain. Annoyingly, the food for your aunt's dog contains the trigger *Bailey* has to avoid. Unlike the happy dog image on the package suggests, giving him this food causes him pain, flatulence, and lethargy; catching a stick will be out of the question for this poor pooch. Maybe, you also imagine your aunt, whose dog feels well, even after consuming what you would never feed him— you remember a cream pie that fell victim to that bitch. "Hogwash!" she would say. "Dogs can eat anything! A dog intolerance? If he only eats enough there will be no farts!"

What is your position at that moment? Back on the couch or driving through the rain to the expert dealer? Now, I am relieved. Therefore, the dog of your friend is worth spending time and money as well as acting considerably. If, at any point it becomes difficult for you to keep your diet, think about the happy *Bailey* and send the square couch potato dog back to your aunt's home!

In the end, I call upon you to take responsibility for your nutrition. Show respect to your body. Acquire the necessary courage and discipline. Your body is a part of you. Just as many vegetarians stand by their dietary choices for the duration of their lives, you should stand by your diet and your body. Be yourself. The key is not starting out perfect, but starting at all and making small improvements every day. That is something you can do! You have the courage and *Bailey* will give you the courage.

Your target should be to change your sustenance day by day, food by food, in such a way as to allow you to lead a mostly symptom-free life. All beginnings are difficult, however, and as you leap the initial hurdles, you will find further motivation and discipline in discovering how much your nutritional changes are paying off for you.

The first step in that direction is to connect that goal with whatever is most important to you in your life. Independent of where your passions lie, you will enjoy them better by gaining more energy and improved wellbeing.

Do you not believe me? The retriever sneaks through the house and as he sees a cat pass by through the window, his only reaction is to fart, then, he retreats into his dog hatchet with an abdominal cramp. Curing the food for aunt's dog that got him into the hot water – you do not want to end up likewise. What about this instead: The retriever sneaks through the house, hears steps, stalks to the open window, stops and sees what looks like a burglar nearby the post box (he does not see the letters in his hands). In a flash, *Bailey* is on the road right behind him giving him a good bark! Pure energy!

What triggers your passion? What is your affair of the heart? Gain strength by keeping a diet that is best for you and give it a fresh start. Turn your attention and abilities toward eating in a way that will help you achieve your goals. If you are uncertain whether you can reach, your goals do this: Imagine that you have already done it. How? Cut out the following card and fold it as indicated. Then put it somewhere you can see it every day. Ideally, you can take a picture of yourself after a particularly fruitful milestone and put it on the drawing. Then let it encourage you to continue improving your nutrition each day. *Stephen William Hawking* has never stopped producing outstanding scientific works despite suffering from a myasthenia. Why? Because he is following his heart and because he has a positive attitude about life. Who seeks excuses when they are passionate about something? When it comes to passion, it is all about the how. It is about doing what is possible and thus it is always all about the solution. There are similar examples in sports. *Melissa Stockwell* achieves first class athletic performance despite having lost a leg. Her sport is her passion, and she finds ways to excel in it regardless of the circumstances life gave her.

So what is your passion? Write it down. Then make it clear to yourself that a symptom-reducing diet will positively affect your achievement. Then get on your way to making this nutrition a part of your life. In addition—always remember about your friend, *Bailey*, the dog.

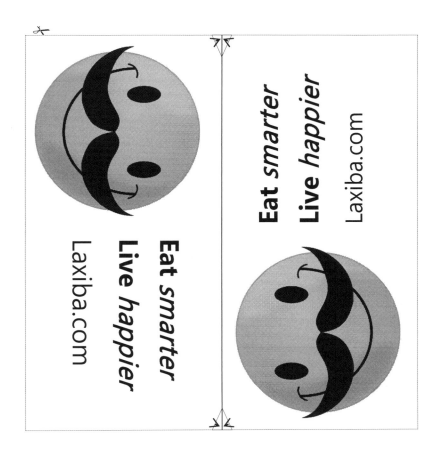

Eat smarter
Live happier
Laxiba.com

Eat smarter
Live happier
Laxiba.com

2.4.2   Mealtimes

Even when and how often you eat can affect your digestion. Who better to ask on that subject than athletes? They, in particular, depend on an optimal nutrient supply. The analysis shows that over 97% of elite Canadian athletes eat at least three times a day; 57% of them also take a snack in the morning, 71% in the afternoon and 58% in the evening. Moreover, regular mealtimes have a positive effect on the cardiovascular system. A study of more than 4,500 children showed that the risk of childhood obesity markedly decreases the more often children eat during the day. How is that? Well, ask the mail carrier of *Bailey's* owner, whether he dares bringing him his letters after eating a gravitationally detrimental meal, his daily ration, in the morning.

2.4.3   Eating out

At home, restricting one's consumption of fructose-containing foods is rather easy. Now you want to eat at a restaurant of a friend's house so what do you do? Of course, you understand that a restaurant staff usually does not have the dietician's expertise required to tell you the ingredients of each meal. Luckily, you can help yourself. For example by learning about some foods that you can usually eat without having to think about them. These include eggs, fish or meat without breading or sauce, kiwis, leafy salads dressed with oil, oregano, pepper and salt, oranges, basil pesto, potatoes, rice, and tortillas. You have to be careful with diabetic products and prepared sauces, as they often contain fructose or sorbitol. What about menus, however? Have you ever spent time at a restaurant considering what the ideal combination of menu items would be for you? The good thing is that you can often ask for a change to menu items without paying extra if you ask the server. You can likewise voice your needs to your hosts when you receive an invitation to a meal. To make it easy, just hand out the safe products list (see Chapter 2.6). You can send it out with the following message, for example:

"Dear [name of the host],

I was glad to receive your invitation to [occasion like your wedding], and I am happy to come. If it is possible for you to cook some of the foods that are included in the attached table separately from the other meals, then I can take part in the meal, as well. Please tell me whether that will be possible so that I can plan accordingly.

Thank you and see you soon!

[Your name]"

The safe products list, see Chapter 2.6, also makes it easier for a restaurant kitchen to find a suitable meal for you. As fast food chains are not as readily equipped to adapt their menus, you will find many fast food chain products and the portion sizes you can stomach in the third part of this book. You can stay on the safe side by always having your book with you. However, it will hardly be always at hand, unlike a foldable list for your purse or wallet. In Chapter 2.5 you will find the cheat sheet for fructose with the tolerable portion sizes of some common products. This list also includes information on fructose and sorbitol names and trigger-free products.

2.4.4   Convenience foods

Unfortunately, fructose is a part of many convenience foods or is naturally contained in the ingredients. However, you will find exceptions, even when shopping on the cheap, including convenience foods that advertise the use of natural ingredients. The cheat sheet (see Chapter 2.5) will inform you, which ingredient on a package mean that the food contains fructose or sorbitol.

2.4.5   Medicine and oral hygiene

Anything you take into your mouth can cause symptoms if it contains fructose. What is more, sorbitol, in particular, is included in many oral hygiene products. An example of a sorbitol-free toothpaste is *JASON® healthy mouth*. Use dental floss without wax, and find a mouthwash such as *TheraBreath® Fresh Breath Oral Rinse*. It sometimes gets tricky, as sorbitol is not always obvious as an ingredient. If you are in doubt, call the customer service hotline of the respective product and ask them for clarification.

The search for sorbitol-free medicines may be especially hard, so ask your pharmacist for assistance. Many nasal sprays, eye drops, and expectorants contain this additive. However, if you look hard enough, you will usually find alternatives for these as well. Examples of sorbitol-free pharmaceuticals include: *Allegra® 12 Hour Allergy* (allergy), *Allerest® PE Allergy & Sinus Relief—Tablets* (frontal sinusitis), *Ayr® Saline Nasal Rinse Kit* (frontal sinusitis), *Florax® DS Diarrhea Relief Vials* (diarrhea), *Hyland's® Earache—Drops* (earache), *Mucinex® 12 Hour Extended Release Expectorant—Tablets* (expectorant), *Mucinex® Sinus-Max Severe Congestion Relief—Tablets* (frontal sinusitis), *SinuCleanse® Neti Pot All Natural Nasal Wash System* (frontal sinusitis) and *Visine-A® Eye Allergy Relief, Antihistamine & Redness Reliever, Drops* (allergy). When considering medicines that contain fructose, take into account the amount you can stomach at your sensitivity, which is 0.5g of fructose at the standard level. It helps to know that middle-sized capsules contain 0.58g at the most, and the largest, 1.6g per piece while tablets are usually even a little lighter. For mixtures, a teaspoon holds about 5 ml/g and a tablespoon 5–15 ml/g.

Despite your best efforts at researching your intolerances, you may find yourself unable to stomach medicine for whatever reason. If you are having symptoms, search for alternatives. If in doubt, use the symptom-test-sheet. Write down your symptoms while using it and compare it with a record of your diet taken when you were not using the medicine, for example, on your efficiency check sheet. You can use any sheet where you recorded your symptoms after refraining from fructose.

2.4.6   Nutritional supplements

If you take vitamin supplements, the following examples are fructose- and sorbitol-free:

Nature's Bounty® Vitamin B-12, 1000mcg, *Nature Made® Vitamin B6 100mg* Dietary Supplement Tablets, *Walgreens® Multivitamin Ultimate Men's Tablets*, *Walgreens® Multivitamin Ultimate Women's Tablets*. A long-term trial did not prove the use of multivitamin supplements. If you take them, make sure not to take too much of certain vitamins. Vitamins that can be unsafe in excess include *B3*, *B6*, as well as *A*, *D*, *E* and *K*, which can cause symptoms of poisoning if you overdose. Thus, you should discuss your intake with your doctor. A viable approach with these vitamins is taking them in three-month cycles. That means taking them for three months and then taking the next three months off.

2.4.7 Protein shakes—nutrition for athletes

There is a partially questionable trend among athletes to take special supplements. If you can cover your protein demand with the products listed in Chapter 2.1.4, you have no need for protein shakes or the like. Many energy bars and electrolyte products contain fructose and sorbitol (see Chapter 3.2). You can often find trigger free alternatives in pharmacies.

2.4.8 Fish and meat

Fish and meat by nature are free of fructose. Nevertheless, you have to be careful with sauce, which may contain fructose or sorbitol. To find out about that, check the list of ingredients of the product.

2.4.9 These actions lead to lasting change

To achieve lasting success, it is important that you monitor your nutrition. If you find yourself starting to ignore the recommended amounts, you should get back on track and restart your commitment as soon as possible. Write down your goal to adapt your nutrition to the stated food and drink portion sizes to reduce abdominal discomfort and improve your quality of life. Stay conscious of the negative consequences of eating "blindly" covered in the first part of this book. Why is it important to change your habits? Re-read your goal and then write down your five most important reasons for striving toward it. Moreover, answer the following question. Why it is important to act **now**?

Probably, you have made the following experience as well. Filled with motivation and enthusiasm you plunge into something, like a New Year's resolution. One goes right after it and even celebrates first successes. However, this feeling trickles away unless soon afterward even bigger successes surpass the first one. If that does not happen, a slight inertia arises. If you change your diet, this can happen to you as well. It is like there is an angel on your one shoulder to whom you say that you are going to keep at it even if it becomes arduous yet there is an imp sitting on your other shoulder, which is already laughing at his sleeve. In fact, the way gets steeper after the first yards. Many then let things slide, which makes further successes impossible, and the symptoms come back. "Isn't that unfair?" the imp is telling you, "you are putting in your effort for days and how does it pay off? You are having the same symptoms as you had before. Let it be." The angel may have screamed so much that it is croaky by now and shrugs his shoulders exhaustedly. "Sorry, but I tried my best," one excuses oneself trying not to look at the grinning devil.

It is a cognitive bias to believe that it is easier just to accept one's symptoms than to change your diet to avoid them. What about you? Did you catch yourself close to giving up? If so, send the devil on your shoulder to the desert where it belongs.

I can promise you: After you changed your diet to fit the food's fructose content, you will have more energy and a higher quality of life. In addition, after you have mastered staying on the right path for some month, you will find that you are getting used to it, which will make it even easier to stick with it. Getting used to it is something that the imp has deliberately concealed: Once you have taken the first pitch, you get accustomed to quickly assessing foods about their content of fructose and learns to notice fructose hideouts. Juggling with the amounts becomes so easy that you do not have to think long. At the start, the cheat sheet and this book will serve you well. Later you no longer need both as you know yourself what is right for you. The imp that you sent to the desert now is hot with anger, and you are the one that has a big grin on the face. You have the best arguments to be tenacious!

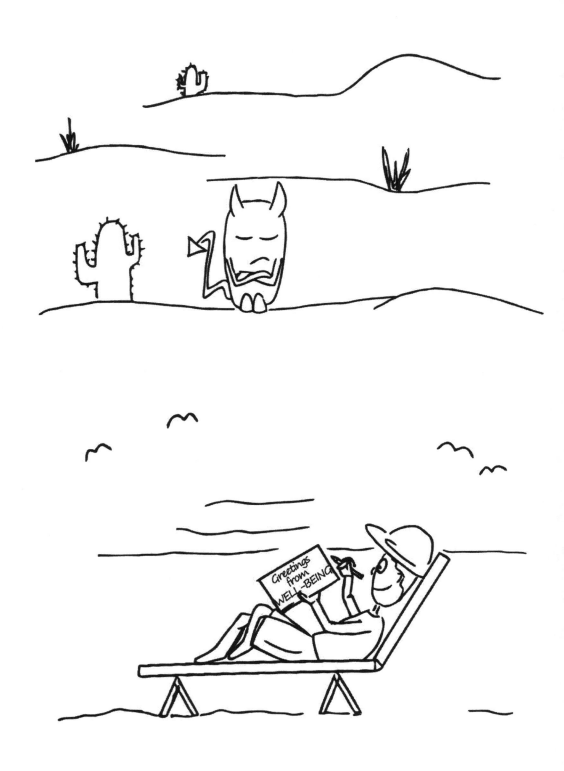

Are you uncertain as to whether you are going to remain motivated? Create an objective agreement with yourself. Note down in writing, why it pays off to you, to endure. Which goal do you want to achieve? For example, like this:

Objective agreement (write it down yourself)

What: comply with the acceptable amounts – Send the devil to the desert.

How to measure it: daily at 7:45 pm (set an alarm on your phone): did I comply with the portion restrictions?

Consequence: YES, you complied, so give yourself a small reward. NO, you did not so do 10 pushups or mow the lawn (anything you can do, which is good for you but you do not like doing).

Get it done: start within three days and keep on actively managing your diet until you have formed a habit of doing it.

Activities: Put this book into your kitchen and the cheat sheet into your wallet; inform those close to you; create reminders in your flat and your car, place your objective agreement somewhere where you can see it at least once a day (e.g. your mirror).

A good way to ensure that you stay committed is to integrate your spouse. Ask them to motivate you and to reflect back to you, which positive changes they notice about you. Another option is to book one of our coaches at *https://laxiba.com/trainer* to help you implement the steps explained in this book. What is more, you will find a way to talk with others and motivate each other at *https://laxiba.com/team.*

The more vivid and multifaceted you can imagine your life after a successful conversion of your diet, the more likely you are to keep moving forward with it and doing what is necessary. Have you been in a rut one day? Forget about it; get the job done better the day after! You can use this book as a compass and correct your course back to being well!

2.4.10 Why fructose and sorbitol are used

Sorbitol makes products free from table sugar to enable diabetics to consume them as well as keeps chocolates moist. For drugs, sorbitol is a carrier for active substances because it is simple and works well. Fructose also can create certain flavours and is often contained in products that contain processed fruits. There would be alternatives that work well in many cases, which would not cost much more. So far, there is no strong lobby against using fructose and sorbitol in foods or making them easier to avoid, yet. Of course, they also occur naturally, but that is not a valid reason to use them instead of the also naturally occurring Stevia in, for example, chewing gums.

2.4.11 Positive aspects of the diet

Do you want to disagree with me after reading the headline? For many the fructose diet equals abdication. In its original sense, however, diet (from the Greek díaita) means "lifestyle" or "way of life." Are abdication and the feeling of a downer an accurate description of the lifestyle that you want? On the contrary, you perform the diet to lower you symptoms and thus increases your quality of life. As you find out, which foods you can eat concerning their fructose content you will automatically start thinking about what you eat in general. The chances are that you will end up eating healthier, and healthy is a much friendlier summary of your lifestyle. Of course, an alternative to the diet would be the use of medicine, like painkillers or drugs to stop diarrhea. Better yet, is to make sure symptoms do not occur in first place. You can also use fructose dissolving enzyme capsulses to achieve the latter aim; they are quite costly though.

2.4.12 Testing yourself

Some of those affected by fructose reportedly struggle to absorb other ingredients like aspartame or maltodextrin. If you have reason to believe that this applies to you, get *THE IBS NAVIGATOR* and follow the alternative introductory diet outlined there.

2.4.13 Sweetener's sorbitol content

Pure stevia is sorbitol-free. Aside from that, sorbitol is contained in many sweeteners as well as light and sugar-free products.

Summary

A healthy, balanced diet, fixed mealtimes, and regular exercise are important not only in case of a fructose intolerance but for all people. Unfortunately, sometimes fructose is included in products although fructose free alternatives are available. Hence, especially when eating convenience foods or taking drugs, watch out for fructose in the ingredients. Stick to the fructose diet if it works. The longer you persist, the easier it gets to maintain it.

2.5   The cheat sheets

C ut out the leaflet on the following page. Please fold it along the thick lines. Start with the dotted line. Then fold it again at the half-dashed line. You can now keep this important information at hand when you are out and about or shopping.

Flyer for fructose intolerance

If you mix fructose with sorbitol-containing products, you tolerate less and if you do, so with glucose containing products you can tolerate more fructose. The identifier number for sorbitol is 420. The following table shows you with which factor you can multiply the fructose amounts when you consume or mix the glucose containing foods with them:

Foods	Portion weight	B x
Avocado (Florida)	37g	2.25
Fresh figs	50g	2.0
Maple syrup	30g	1.5
Mozzarella	28g	1.25
Sweet corn	82g	3.25
Thin slice of pineapple	56g	2.25

Foods that contain fructose:

- Cereals with fructose syrup and HFCS
- Many convenience foods
- Canning sugar, honey and corn syrup
- Some sweeteners
- Most fruits also, when they are dry
- Many soft drinks, fruits, and alcoholic beverages
- Some sauces

Foods that contain sorbitol:

- Fruits, juices and alcoholic beverages
- Products for athletes like protein bars
- Convenience foods and sauces
- chewing gum and mints other than those that only contain stevia and table sugar
- Light und isotonic drinks
- Drugs and oral hygiene products
- Diabetics and dietary products
- Chocolates, cream, and cakes

LAXIBA®

Fructose intolerance serving sizes

Pineapple ¾ P; 140g
Apple ☒
Apricot ☺+¾ P/E; 35g
Balsamic vinegar ☺
Banana ☺+¼ P/E; 118g
Blueberry. muffin. 26 E; 110g
Beer ☺
Big Mac® 5 E; 215g
Bitter lemon ☒
Pears ½ C; 15g
Lettuces 1¼ P; 85g
Cauliflower ☺

Broccoli 3 P; 85g
Blackberries 1¾ P; 140g
Cranberries ☺
Cinnamon crumble
GoLEAN ☺+¼ P; 30g
Coca Cola® ½ G; 200ml
Corn flakes ☺+1½ P/P; 30g
Strawberries ½ P; 140g
Special K® Original ☺
Garden salad 8¼ P; 85g
Ginger Ale ☒2 G; 200ml
Cucumber 4¾ E; 85g
Oatmeal ☺

Raspberries ½ P; 140g
Honey ¼ P 21g
Chicken sweet'n sour 2½T15g
Currants 1 P; 140g
Coffee ☺
Potatoes ☺
Chewing gum ☺
Ketchup ☺+¼ P/T; 15g
Cherries 1 P; 140g
Kiwi 1 E; 86g
Cabbage ☺+¾ P/P; 85g
Pumpkin butternut ☺
Long Island Ice tea ¾ G; 200ml
M & M's® ☺
Mango 1 T; 15g
Mate tea ☺
Melon 1¾ T; 15g
Milk ☺
Granola bar ½ E; 30g
Nectarines ¾ E; 142g
Oranges 2¼ E; 140g

Pepper ½ P; 85g
Pepsi® ½ G; 200ml
Peach ☺+½ P/E; 140g
Plum ☺+¼ P/E; 15g
Mushrooms ☺
Pizza ☺
Red Bull® ☺+7P/G; 200ml
Rice ☺
Sauerkraut ☺
Chocolate ☺
Champagne ☺
Smacks® ☺+12 P/P; 30g
Sushi 16 P; 140g
Tomatoes 3 P; 85g
Tonic Water® ☒2 G; 200ml
Grapes ¼ P; 140g
Wine ¾ G; 200ml
Wheat bread ¾ E; 42g
Whopper® 2¾ E; 315g
Lemon ☺
7UP® ☒2 G; 200ml

Portion unit abbreviations:

Exemplar	Cup	Glass	Portion	Tbsp.
E	C	G	P	T

☒=avoid; ☺=nearly free; ☺=is free of it ☺+=free and contains glucose: B-factor: B-factor/per unit

Front **Flyer sorbitol intolerance**

Tolerated in case of sorbitol intolerance are

Maltodextrin	Sorbic acid	Barley malt syrup
Sodium sorbate	Potassium sorbate	Calcium sorbate
Sorbitan…	Polyoxyethylene(20)-sorbitan…	

(INS add. numbers: 200-203, 432-436, 491-495)

These ingredients are sugar alcohols:

Sorbitol	Mannitol	Xylitol	
Lactitol	(Ethyl-) Maltol	Hexanhexol	
Glucitol	Maltitol/-syrup	Inositol	
Isomalt	Palatinit®	Sionon	
Erythritol	Pinitol		

(INS add. numbers: 420-21, 636-37, 953, 965-7)

Hence, avoid foods that contain them.

Back **Sugar alcohols like sorbitol are often contained in:**

- Diabetics and dietary products
- Athletes products and energy bars
- Convenience foods and sauces
- Chewing gum and mints except for those that only contain stevia and table sugar
- Some light and isotonic beverages
- Drugs and mouthwashes

- Bars, chocolates, cream, and cream pies
- Moreover, some fruits, their juices, and alcoholic beverages as well as some vegetables

Interior left **Sorbitol intolerance portion sizes**

Pineapple ¾ P-140g	Broccoli ☺
Apple ☺² E; 182g	Blackberries ☺² P-140g
Apricots ¾ E; 35g	Cranberries 45¼ P-55g
Vinegar balsa. 23 P-15g	Froot Loops® ☺
Banana 9¼ E; 118g	Coca Cola® ☺
Blueberry Muffin 88 E; 113g	Corn Flakes ☺ P-30g
	Strawberries ¼ P-140g
Beer 10 G-200ml	Special K® original ☺
Big Mac® 6½ E; 215g	Garden salad 16 P-85g
Bitter Lemon ☺	Ginger Ale ☺
Pear ¼ E; 15g	Cucumber 1 E; 85g
Lettuces 3 P-85g	Oats ☺
Cauliflower 2½ P-85g	

Interior right

Chicken sweet and sour ☺	Peppers ☺ E; 85g
Raspberries 1½ P-140g	Pepsi® ☺ G-200ml
Honey 1¾ T; 15g	Peach ¼ E; 140g
Currants 2½ P-140g	Plum ¾ T; 15g
Coffee ☺	Mushroom ¾ T; 15g
Potatoes 45¼ P-110g	Pizza ¾ E; 209g
Ketchup 3¾ T; 15g	Red Bull® ☺
Cherries ¼ T; 15g	Rice ☺
Kiwi ☺	Sauerkraut ¾ T; 15g
Cabbage 58¾ P-85g	Chocolate 48 P-25g
Pumpkin butternut ☺	Champaign ¾ G-200ml
Long Island Icet. 16 G-200ml	Smacks® 83¼ P-30g
M & M's® ☺	Sushi 1½ P-140g
Mango 4 T; 15g	Tomatoes 1 T; 85g
Mate tea ☺	Grapes ½ P-140g
Mayonnaise ☺	Wine ¾ G-200ml
Melon 14¼ P-140g	Wheat bread 26¼ P-42g
Milk ☺	Whopper® 1 E; 315g
Granola bar ☺²	Lemon ☺
Nectarines 1 T; 15g	Chewing gum light ☺
Oranges ☺ E; 140g	7UP® ☺

If you are sensitive avoid any food but one with ☺

Portion unit abbreviations (gram follows):

Exemplar	Cup	Glas	Portion	Tbsp.
E	C	G	P	T

⊗=avoid; ☺=nearly free; ☺=is free of it

Cheat sheet content

If you have a fructose intolerance, be mindful of fructose and HFCS while reading the ingredient lists. As you learned before, sorbitol lowers the amount of fructose-containing products you can tolerate. To determine sorbitol-free products, however, you, unfortunately, have to navigate an unbelievable minefield of identifiers, despite the high prevalence of the condition. As I am unaware of studies that tested, if the interaction with fructose is limited to sorbitol, I will show you the names of the other sugar alcohols as well:[1]

Caution... these products contain fructose:

- Cereals with high fructose corn syrup (HFCS) or isoglucose, glucose-fructose syrup, fructose-glucose syrup and high fructose maize syrup. Unless they are listed in the food tables of this book you cannot know how much you can tolerate of them
- Many convenience foods
- Preserving sugar
- Honey and corn syrup (fructose quantity is unclear)
- Some sweeteners
- Many fruits, dried fruits, juices, and alcoholic drinks
- Many soft drinks

These prodcuts often contain Sugar alcohols like sorbitol:

- Diabetic and dietary products
- Electrolyte products and energy bars
- Convenience foods and prepared sauces
- Chewing gums and mints, except those sweetened only with Stevia, for example. Sorbitol is either only contained in traces or not contained at all in Wrigley's® Spearmint, Doublemint and Juicy Fruit
- Some "light," i.e., sugar-free, and isotonic beverages
- Medicine and oral hygiene products
- Bars, pralines, sweet pastries, tarts, prepared cream
- Puréed, pickled or breaded sausages, fish, and meat

---

[1] There is an immediate need for simplification here. A proper solution is the declaration "contains sorbitol".

Noncritical ingredients concerning sorbitol[2]

Maltodextrin	Sorbic acid	Barley malt syrup
Sodium sorbate	Potassium sorbate	Calcium sorbate
Sorbitan...	Polyoxyethylene (20) –sorbitan-...	

Sugar alcohol names[3]

Sorbitol	Mannitol	Xylitol
Lactitol	(Ethyl-) Maltol	Hexanhexol
Glucitol	Maltitol/-syrup	Inositol
Isomalt	Palatinit®	Sionon
Erythritol	Pinitol	

---

[2] INS additive numbers: 200–203, 432–436, 491–495.
[3] INS additive numbers: 420–21, 636–37, 953, 965–67.

2.6   The safe products list

L ikely, if you yourself do not have a fructose intolerance, someone in your circle of acquaintances has the irritable bowel syndrome or an intolerance towards some ingredient. As a good host, you may have already been in a situation to consider those to make sure that none of your guests encounters an uneasy feeling after an invitation.

If you ask your guests to tell you about any problematic ingredient you should accustom to, you are prepared professionally: Such a question will always leave a positive impression as it shows that your guest's well-being is important to you. You are well accustomed to any guest, if you make sure that some foods that are usually tolerable for anyone are on the menu. How can you achieve that? It is quite simple: make sure to offer the sauces separately from the side dishes. Hence, provide a bowl of potatoes, another bowl with butter, a third one with salad and lastly one with dressings. By the way, with some exceptions like garlic and onions anyone can tolerate most herbs and spices. The table on the following page shows you some usually safe foods.

Fruit	Vegetables	Warm dishes
Blackberries	Avocado, green	Brandy vinegar
Currants	Basil	Caviar
Dates, fresh	Chard	Chinese oyster sauce
Figs, fresh	Chives	Fish, meat, shrimp and
Goji berries	Coriander	shellfish*
Lemon zest	Green peppers	Kraft® Italian Dressing
Loganberry	Horseradish	
Papaya	Kelp	Kraft® Mayonnaise
Passion fruit	Oregano	Oils
Rhubarb	Parsnips	Kraft® Thousand Island
	Peppermint, fresh	Dressing®
	Rice	Pepper and salt
	Rosemary	Rice bread
	Rutabaga	Rice noodles
	Squash: Butternut, cala-bash, giant and spaghetti	Soy oil
	Thyme	Spelt flour
	Yam	Tabasco® sauce

*Non pureed and without breading and sauce.

Beverages		Other
Black coffee	Baking powder	Pecan nuts
Brandy	Brazil nuts	Pine nuts
Gin	Brown sugar	Pistachios
Jasmine tea	Cashews	Pumpkin seeds
Maté tea	Coconut	Rice bread
Peppermint tea	Gelatin	Spelt
Rum	Ginkgo	Walnuts
Tequila	Licorice	White sugar
Tonic Water	Macadamia nuts	
Vodka	Maple syrup	
Water	Peanut butter	
Whiskey	Peanuts	

2.7 Recipes

2.7.1 Apricot cuts

Tolerable amount concerning the fructose content: as much as you like

What you need:

4 tbsp. of apricot jam
4/5 cup of dried, fine sliced apricots
One cup of butter
One cup of flour (in case of celiac disease, use gluten free flour)
3/5 cup of rice flour
One tsp. of vanilla-extract
2/5 cup of sugar, as well as some to dust over

Preparation:

Preheat the oven at 390 °F top and bottom heat or 360 °F convection heat. Then, lay out an eight in deep backing tray with baking paper. Now add the apricots and jam in a small pan with 4 tbsp. water. Simmer over medium heat until they are thick. Then squash the apricots a little with a fork and let them cool down. Add the butter, vanilla extract and sugar in a bowl and mix with the blender. Afterward, add the rice flour and the flour and whip with a spoon or your hands to form a dough. Then, divide the dough into two equal pieces. Spread one-half of the dough on the baking sheet. Knead the remaining dough into an eight in² square piece and place it on top. Press alongside the edge of the dough and stab some small holes into it with a fork. Bake for 25-30 minutes until the corners turn golden. Leave it in the baking mold for the cool down and sprinkle powdered sugar over it. Slice three cuts to the top and the sides and that is it.

2.7.2 Banana cake

Tolerable amount concerning the fructose content: 15 pieces

What you need:

Two ripe bananas
A handful of banana chips
One packet of baking powder (celiac disease? Use gluten-free baking powder)
3/5 cup of butter and something for the baking mold
Two large eggs
1/5 cup of icing
3/5 cup of flour (use gluten free flour if gluten intolerant)
3/5 cup of sugar

Preparation:

Preheat the oven to 390 °F top and bottom heat or 360 °F circulating air. Meanwhile spread some butter into a marble cake mold. Gently mix the butter and sugar together. Then slowly add the eggs and some flour. Afterward, stir the rest of the flour, baking powder and bananas into the mix. Place the dough in a baking mold and bake the cake for about 30 minutes until it well rises. Now let it cool down in the mold for about 10 minutes. Following, prepare the frosting with two teaspoons of water, douse the cake with it and decorate with the banana chips.

2.7.3   Creamy rice pudding

Tolerable amount concerning the fructose content: as much as you like

What you need (for four servings):

One tbsp. butter

2/5 cup of cranberries

One egg

3/5 cup of rice

2 cups of rice milk

One pinch of salt

½ tsp. of vanilla extract

¼ cup of sugar

Preparation:

Cook the rice in water. Then add 350g of cooked rice with ¾ of the milk, the sugar and a pinch of salt in a new pan, stir from time to time and let the mix cook for another 3 minutes. Meanwhile, beat the egg in a small bowl with a wire whisk. At the end of the cooking time, add to the mix with the rest of the milk and the cranberries and let it simmer it yet another 3 minutes. It is important that you always stir it. Now remove the pan from the plate and mix with the butter and the vanilla extract - Bon appetite.

2.7.4   Kiwi sauce (e.g. with ice)

Tolerable amount concerning the fructose content: one and ½ servings

What you need (one serving):

Three tsp. of maple syrup
Two ripe green kiwi fruits
Two tsp. of lime or lemon juice

Preparation:

Peel the kiwis, dice them and blend them afterwards together with the lime or lemon juice. If you love pure green, sieve out the remaining black seeds later on.

2.7.5 Fruit salad

Tolerable amount concerning the fructose content: as much as you like

What you need (four servings):

4/5 cup of pineapple
One banana, ½ cup
One cup of strawberry
One orange, 3/5 cup
One cup of cranberries
One tbsp. of lemon juice

Preparation:

Peel the pineapple, remove the stem and cut into finger-thick pieces. Now peel the orange, remove the seeds and chop up, also cut the strawberries. Place the pieces in a bowl and pour the lemon juice over them. Stir well now and you did it. If you suffer from a fructose intolerance, it is better if you blend the salad and make sorbet, because your tolerance depends on the glucose content of the cranberries.

2.7.6   Fruit salad with curd

Tolerable amount concerning the fructose content: as much as you like

What you need (eight servings):

Maple syrup
Two cups of canned pineapple (if fresh the curd turns bitter)
One and ¼ cup of cranberries
One and ¼ cup of canned mandarins
Two cups of sour cream or cottage cheese with a little milk

Preparation:

Cut the pineapple into finger-thick pieces. Now place the fruit and sour cream in a bowl. After stirred well, season well with the maple syrup. To consume enough glucose-containing cranberries, puree the fruits with a blender.

2.7.7 Lemon bar

Tolerable amount concerning the fructose content: ~30 pieces

What you need:
For the dough:

3/5 cup of butter
¾ cup of flour (celiac disease? Use gluten free flour)
One tbsp. milk
1/5 cup of rice flour
4/5 cup of brown sugar

For the topping:

Three eggs
2 tbsp. of flour (celiac disease? Use gluten free flour)
Icing sugar
The zest of three lemons
4/5 cup of ml lemon juice
4/5 cup of sugar

Preparation:

Preheat the oven at 430 °F top and bottom heat or 390 °F air circulation. Cover a 9 in. baking tray with baking paper. Mix the butter, the flour, rice flour and sugar in a bowl, until only small lumps form. Then add the milk and spread the dough on the baking tray. Let it bake for 17 minutes until golden brown. Then remove the tray and reduce the oven temperature to 390 °F top and bottom heat or 360 °F air circulation. Whisk the lemon juice and the eggs, the sugar, the flour and the lemon zest in a bowl. Pour this concentrate over the dough and bake the lemon bars for another 15 minutes until the surface almost firm. Let it cool down on the tray. Finally, cut and powder - ready to enjoy.

2.7.8   Orange-peppermint-salad

Tolerable amount concerning the fructose content: two and ¼ servings

What you need (for four servings)**:**

12 pitted dates, cut lengthwise
Four oranges
A small bunch of mint: some leaves finely cut and a few left a whole
One tbsp. of water

Preparation:

Peel the orange and place it together with the liberated juice in a bowl. Afterward, add the date pieces and the chopped peppermint leaves to the water and mix gently. Finally, top it with whole mint leaves.

2.7.9   Pancakes

Tolerable amount concerning the fructose content: depends on your filling

What you need:

One egg
Half a cup of flour (celiac disease? Use gluten free flour)
1 and ¼ cup of rice milk
Sunflower oil

Preparation:

Put the flour into a bowl and make a hole in the middle, in which you put the egg together with the rice milk. Now whisk everything well with a mixer. Add a quarter of the rice milk and continue to add the rest once the batter is lump free. Now let the dough rest and after 20 minutes whisk it again. Preheat a small non-stick frying pan and pour the oil into it. Cover the whole bottom of the pan with a thin layer of dough. Fry the pancakes on each side, until golden brown. Place some baking paper between the pancakes when you pile them, so they remain crispy. Serve with any filling.

2.7.10 Pizza dough

Tolerable amount concerning the fructose content: as much as you like

What you need:

7g (one filled tsp) yeast (celiac disease? Use dry gluten-free yeast. First, let it rise with a tsp. of sugar in a cup that is half-full of water. After that, mix it with the rest of the water and flour. Often, it takes some time until the dough has risen.)
One and ½ cups of flour (celiac disease? Use gluten-free flour, here you may have to experiment a bit)
One 1/5 cups of water

Preparation:

Put the flour with a tsp. salt, yeast and 275 ml lukewarm water in a bowl and mix everything for about 5 minutes to form a dough. Now, take out the dough and let it rise it in a lightly oiled bowl until it rises about twice the size. Knead the dough afterwards for a bit, then cut it in half and roll out each of both parts on a thin layer of flour as thin as possible. Now garnish the pizza as desired and bake in the oven at 430 °F air circulation.

2.7.11 Rhubarb, roasted

Tolerable amount concerning the fructose content: as much as you like

What you need (five servings):
1 and 1/3 cup of Rhubarb
1/3 cup of brown sugar

Preparation:
Preheat the oven at 390 °F top and bottom heat or 360 °F air circulation. Wash the Rhubarb then shake off the water. Cut the end and the middle of the sticks into small finger-sized pieces. Cover a closed baking tray with a baking sheet and spread the Rhubarb on it. Sprinkle some sugar over it and cover the Rhubarb with it. Bake the Rhubarb for about 15 minutes with baking paper on top. Then remove the baking paper and shake the plate slightly. Then continue baking for about five minutes. When the Rhubarb is ready, it is soft, but not mushy.

2.7.12 Rhubarb cake

Tolerable amount concerning the fructose content: as much as you like

What you need:

One packet of baking powder (celiac disease? Use gluten-free baking powder)
Four large eggs
One cup of flour (celiac disease? Use gluten free flour)
Icing sugar
Pre-roasted Rhubarb, as described before.
One cup of sweet cream butter and even something for the baking tray
One tsp. vanilla extract
3/5 cup of custard
One cup of brown sugar

Preparation:

First, prepare the roasted Rhubarb and drain the juice. Preheat now the oven at 390 °F top and bottom heat or 180 degrees air circulation. Wipe a nine in cake springform pan with butter. Put 3 tbsp. of the vanilla pudding in a separate bowl. The rest you whisk up creamy with butter, the flour, baking powder, eggs and sugar in a bowl. Pour one-third of the mix in the cake form and place about half of the Rhubarb over it. Put one more third of dough over this layer and flatten it as smooth as possible. Cover the top with the rest of the Rhubarb and pour the remaining mixture over it, this time, the surface remains rough. Then use the remaining 3 tbsp. of the vanilla pudding to place on top. Bake the cake for 40 minutes, until it rises and becomes golden. Cover it with baking paper and leave it baking for another 15 minutes. The cake is ready when you stab it with a toothpick, and it comes out clean. Sprinkle some icing sugar over the cake after it cooled down.

2.7.13 Rhubarb-smoothie

Tolerable amount concerning the fructose content: as much as you like

What you need (for two servings):

One small banana
One cup of cranberry juice
2/5 cup of frozen Rhubarb
Five tbsp. (1/2 cups) of vanilla yogurt

Preparation:

Cut the banana into small pieces and puree everything together in a blender.

2.7.14 Tropical fruit salad

Tolerable amount concerning the fructose content: ½ portion

What you need (six servings):
One and 2/3 cups of pieced cantaloupe
Two peeled kiwis
One and 2/3 cups of lychees
Three peeled oranges
Two stalks of lemongrass
1/3 cup of brown sugar

Preparation:
Cut the lemon grass into pieces and crush it with a rolling pin. Peel the lychees and remove the seeds, catch the juice. Mix the juice with the sugar and the lemongrass and heat it up for about a minute in a pan until the sugar has melted. Then let the broth cool down and sprinkle it over the fruits.

2.8 Stress management

Stress can affect your stomach and worsen fructose intolerance symptoms. Hence, it is important to reduce it. To find out its effect on you, fill out your symptom-test-sheet on a day when you have a lot of stress. Developing a solution-oriented way to manage your worries can help you do so. How does that help? The more you stress over something, the more brain areas that you need for a reasonable decision are being set off. The body does so, because, in a certain way, our bodies are prepared for an earlier historical era. Dangerous situations like an attack by a wolf pack left us with three options: fight, flight or playing dead. If we spent too much time thinking in such a situation, it was game over! Hence, we are poled to stop thinking as soon as we feel we are in danger—which is not always helpful in our modern time.

If nowadays your boss storms into your office with some tricky and pressing demands of a huge client, neither a spontaneous attack nor jumping out of the window or acting as dead will be recommendable. Seriously, nowadays usually much different factors trigger stress than it was a few thousand years ago. Aside from noise, extreme temperatures, and air pollution, it is especially the feeling of losing control in a situation, which feels threatening to us. Fear can grab you, when a project is particularly delicate and important, something fundamental has to change, and you are under time pressure.

At the advent of fear, the release of hormones supports fight and flight reactions that enable us to make quick, even if ill-conceived, decisions. Everything inside of you screams "Do something immidiately, no matter what!" Large parts of our brain are set aside for that purpose. You feel stress and tend to make impulsive rather than rational decisions. The hormones lead to a shut down of vast areas of your brain at that moment; you feel stress. The third option your mind conceives in a dangerous situation, playing dead, somewhat corresponds to the extreme modern-day phenomena that is widely known as burnout.

So you have the impulses of a Stone Age hunter but the tasks of a top manager: how can you make that fit together? The only option you have to resist your impulse is to take command of your body and mind. To react appropriately, you are required not to have your hormones to turn off your resources for rational decision-making.

Once your body feels in danger, it is a challenge to halt the rolling wheel of your body's emergency reactions abruptly. Hence, the best thing you can do is to prevent these stress reactions from evolving in the first place. Yoga and progressive muscle relaxation before work are useful stress preventers. Using such techniques before going to work is sensible, as it is seldom possible to take an hour off during the workday. Breaks and disruptions during your working hours are also **counterproductive** if you are dealing with complex tasks; they often lead to poor decisions, more stress, and a short temper. Thus, try to avoid disruption when dealing with sophisticated tasks. You will agree if you imagine working on a complex calculation while your phone is ringing and your colleague enters to chat with you and a technician wanting to maintain your printer is waiting in front of the door. Therefore, try to avoid distractions when you are dealing with challenging tasks.

However, interruptions of simple mental or physical labor lasting a few minutes, rather than seconds, result in slight positive effects. Taking breaks from hard physical labor, meanwhile, show even stronger benefits, lowering the risk of injuries and enhancing endurance. You do not want to be following a printer printing during your break. To make the best use of it, close your eyes and focus on your breathing. Whenever thoughts come up, focus your whole attention bad on your breath without evaluating the thoughts. What makes this better is counting the times that you breathe out and feeling your breath leave your mouth.

Still, relaxation alone might not be the solution. Often, you can identify general worries that effect your mood. So how do you deal with such concerns? Many try to evade them by trying to ignore them, distract themselves or even take alcohol or other supposed comforters. Instead of bringing you closer to your goal, such a reaction, makes matters worse in most cases. The only thing that will help you resolve your troublesome thoughts is actively dealing with them. Only if you can name them, you can find solutions. Also, consider this; ignorance may well be one of the leading causes of failure.

Of course, for most worries no one hands you the solution on a silver platter. You have to take action. An open examination of your concerns and the right strategy can lead you towards a feasible solution. There is an immediate positive effect of this, independent from what solution you find: you avoid panic actions that one tends to in charged situations. If you regularly call a spade a spade and rationally seek solutions to situations you worry about you reduce the number of poor decisions.

By doing so, you can even use your fears—through the process of conquering them—to help you become more successful in your everyday life. What I recommend you do is sit down at a quiet desk at the beginning or end of the day. Next, think about what you are worried about right now and which steps you need to take to prevent the feared outcomes.

It is helpful to create an Excel spreadsheet for doing so or to purchase the standardized and printer-optimized edition at *www.Laxiba.com*. If you want to create the table by yourself, call the first sheet "Worries" and the second one "Task List." Next, write down the following task headings in the first spreadsheet: "Current Worries," "Preventive Measure A," "Preventive Measure B" and "Preventive Measure C." Then enter the following column titles in the second spreadsheet: "Task," "Priority," "Deadline," "Who does it?" and "Done."

You should write down your concerns in the first column of the first sheet. Then, think about what you will need to do to prevent these worries from becoming a reality. Think of three alternatives for each outcome. Enter these into the "Preventive Measure A–C" fields next to each worry, A being the action you want to take first. Then, transfer "Preventive Measure A" to the "Task List" sheet. Next, prioritize the tasks by employing an adapted version of the "Eisenhower method," an organization technique that takes importance and urgency into account, from A to E:

Task is important	**A** *ction now*	**B** *etter do it soon*
Task is unimportant	**C** *hance to do the task if you completed all A and B duties.*	**D** *ull moment task*
E *fface, don't do task*	Task is urgent	Postponable task

In the order from A to D, you then execute your duties on a daily basis. The category E is for tasks that are ineffective and therefore, you leave it. Hence, you prevent worrying and free yourself from doubting whether you are currently doing the right thing. After assessing the tasks from A to D, you fill out the column "Deadline," into which you enter the date at which you want to accomplish the task. Furthermore, you either note "I" or the name of the person that you want to delegate the work to in the column "Who does it?" Finally, you tick off the cell in the column „Done", when you have finished the task.

Another important aspect is keeping your life balanced. A fulfilled family life and friendships also help to improve your stress resistance. To name an example: taking a healthy exercise is beneficial for all areas of your life. Brought to an extreme, though, let's say if you spend ten hours per day at a fitness center, this will take too much of your time away from your other areas—unless you are a personal trainer. The four quadrants of your life are like the four legs of a stool you sit on. Let us call it your life-stool. If each leg is just as long as the others and all are adequately thick, you will sit well and safe. In however you chop off some from one or more legs repeatedly and strengthen another leg, you will start to waggle—until at some point, there is a crack, and you land on your patoot. You have to avoid this "breakdown". Of course, I know that this is exactly the dilemma that burdens many people nowadays. You feel that you have to perform continuously in all areas. Fathers do not only have to work. They also have to spend time with their family. They ought to bring their children to the violin tuition. Then in the evening, they should foster their social contacts and engage in the summer festival of their city. Having a well-trained body is necessary for many. On top of that, you ideally are relaxed and well groomed. For woman and mothers, the expectations are just as high. They feel like they have to perform like men at work and still manage their family, organize the spare time and stay fit. Expectations appear to rise everywhere.

So do not get me wrong: keeping your life in a healthy balance means finding the **right** balance between those things that are important to you personally. It is not about which expectations others have concerning your life's quadrants! It is not about what the society expects from you. What is important is that you consider the key aspects of your individual life. In the table below these are work, relaxation, family and spare time. For you, the quadrants may be different. You set the priorities yourself. Free yourself as much as possible from the influence of the acknowledgment by others, follow the saying "great horses jump tight" and develop a healthy self-confidence and composure.

Instead of delivering an over-the-top performance in one area but lousy results in all others, you want to do at least a satisfying job in all sectors, to remain capable in the end. Which of the family, spare time, relaxation and work quadrants are important is up to you, along with the results you are aiming for with them, such as spending time with those closest to you, taking daily walks, pursuing your hobbies and getting your work done properly. Furthermore, it is important to resist basing your success on external measures. You should nourish a healthy self-confidence and serenity in yourself. Thus, you need to know when finished the task you are doing well enough. Some people get into time trouble because they over deliver on some tasks and then have little time left to take care of other important tasks, which then causes stress. Often it takes 80% of the time to improve on the last 20% of a job, so it pays off if you know if the last 20% are worth it.

Family:	**Relaxation:**
Spend time with those closest to you	Go out for a walk on a daily basis
Spare time:	**Work:**
Pursue your hobbies regularly	Get your work done properly

You can measure your progress about the four quadrants on a monthly basis on a scale of 1 (very good) to 7 (very poor). Always assign 7 points to the area that you are happiest with and other numbers to the remaining quadrants in relation to that one. Afterward, consider whether you want to make any changes to how you are approaching these areas of your life and how you can make those changes. You can also use the spreadsheet you created to manage your worries.

One final point on the topic of stress, even if it may seem trivial: be mindful of your mood, and try to stay upbeat! What you need to do that depends on you. Your mood only partially depends on circumstances. Sometimes simply deciding to be in a good mood can do more than most people realize. Everyone has a load of problems to carry, and it is easier to take it if you commit yourself to a positive outlook.

Do things that excite you as often as possible. Perform activities that contribute to what is most important to you. Is it your family? Then plan an excursion with your family! Is it a sport? Then ask someone to go jogging with you, for example. Consciously take the time to do those things that are close to your heart. Maybe you now object that you do not have time for that and that such self-serving activities would only lead to more stress. Try it out! I bet this qualitatively precious time will not incur losses but help you to mount every day with more tranquility. Plan your activities around what is most important to you in your life. What that means is obviously personal to you! It is your treasure, per se, so you have to dig it out yourself. *Abraham Lincoln* had this to say, to send you on your way: "That some achieve great success is proof to all that others can achieve it as well."

⊛ Summary

Stress can foster fructose intolerance symptoms. Increase your resistance to stress by training to use relaxation techniques, naming fears and worries, developing and noting down solution strategies and adding priorities to them. Make sure you keep your life in the right balance by trading-off between the areas that are important to you. Keep your eye on your goal.

2.9   General summary

1. What you are dealing with

If you have a fructose intolerance, then fructose in food can irritate your gut. The symptoms occur because of your body's limited capacity to absorb fructose before it reaches your large intestine, where it causes the discomforts. A fructose intolerance is often chronic but does not cause cancer. In most cases, following a fitting diet reduces the symptoms to an acceptable level.

2. Are you a unique case?

According to the *World Gastroenterology Organisation (WGO)*, up to one billion people have a dietary intolerance or IBS around the globe. In a way, you are lucky, as you can use this book to help you to reduce your symptoms.

3. Good reasons to follow this diet

An intolerance accompanies you for a long time, maybe for the rest of your life. If the diet works, it is far cheaper than medical treatment and sometimes even more efficient. Many medicines also have side effects. If the diet works for you, it will also lead to a general improvement in your wellbeing. You should find that you are ill less often, better able to concentrate, better at fulfilling social obligations, stronger at sports—your new diet can even enhance your love life!

4. Why you want to take the level test

Sensitivities differ in their severity. The fewer dietary restrictions you face, the more you save yourself the effort and can enjoy a more varied selection of food.

5. What you should pay attention to for the diet

Two things: First, adhere to your portion sizes, which you find in the tables in Chapter 3. Thus, only eat as much of fructose containing foods as your enzyme workers can handle. You should keep eating fructose-containing foods in tolerable amounts, as fruits contain healthy vitamins. Second, eat in a balanced way see Chapter 2.1.4.

6. Dealing with setbacks

You have decided to change your diet and have made the first steps in that direction. Now, you have to stick to it. Moreover, that means to assess properly short-term setbacks. Rebounds are a part of any change process. What is important is that you get back up! The experience of meeting success after facing a blow will strengthen you immensely and ensure that you will be able to get back up even faster next time around. At some point, your experiences and successes will make it a habit for you to persevere and stick to your diet.

It may help you to set a time each Sunday to fill out the symptom test sheet—independent of the other tests. Doing this will remind you of your goal and let you break down the necessary steps toward it on a weekly basis. What is also important is that you become aware of the hurdles you will face. It will be hard to restrict yourself concerning the consumption of some foods that you have come to love. Particularly at the beginning, it will be unnerving to ask for dietary considerations as a dinner guest. Your nutrition plan will be new to others; you may feel criticized for your insistence on maintaining your new eating habits. Explain that you need to do it for the sake of your health. At the same time, express your appreciation for others' support. Moreover, try not giving dietary advice unless someone asks you for it — respecting the eating habits of others. They are more likely to accept yours in turn.

The adversary left for you to face is not standing next to you at the buffet and believes to know better what you can consume. The best captains are always standing ashore. The adversary is in your head and regularly cries "do it as you did it before. Before it was easier!" The influence of our old habits is often greater than we think. After a few days of tenacity, this caller has his big appearance. As soon, as our vigilance is lower he whispers in our ear "This is how you have always done it, and it has always been good, everything else is too exhaustive for you. Simply, show your adversary your weekly symptom test sheet--it works like garlic against vampires. It is the best mean to get rid of old habits, and form new ones! If you always readjust your heading—your diet to your goal, you will come close to it in the end. If you proceed like that, you have a good chance to win against the trigger and old habit imp.

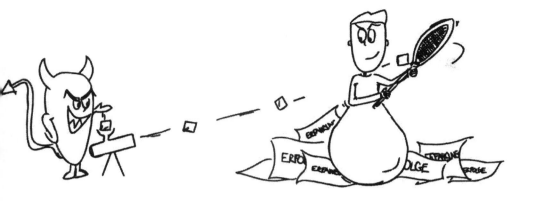

7. FAQs

What do you recommend concerning the diet? Drink at least 1.5 L of water every day. Eat a variety of foods. Even if you are fructose intolerant, try to eat as many fruits as you can to ensure a natural supply of vitamins. It is ok to eat foods that contain fructose; they can even be good for you as long as you keep within your restrictions. The latter does not apply to people with a hereditary fructose intolerance. To do even more for your health, work out regularly.

What can you do if a drink contains too much of fructose to drink a regular glass full? By diluting it with water, you can multiply your tolerable portion. Another option is to take the required number of enzyme capsules for fructose intolerance.

How can you save on cooking time? Cook larger portion sizes. Usually, it only takes a little longer than preparing small ones, and warming the food up is quick. You can keep rice and potatoes in the fridge for days, for instance. Purchase lockable glass containers to store your food keeping it fresh longer.

I have acute symptoms, what can I do? Take a walk and drink up to three liters of drinking water per day.

8. The LAXIBA® quickie

Avoid apple and peach juices and drink orange juice instead, for example. Be careful with sweet non-alcoholic beverages.

Do not start any diet without a proper diagnosis in advance. If you want to do something for your health, in general, stick to the advice see the Chapters starting on pages 39 and 77.

FEEDBACK

Congratulations, you have mastered the background and strategy chapter. Around the globe, the brand *LAXIBA* represents an improved quality of life in connection with abdominal diseases and stress. Our goal is to offer you scientific solutions that you can implement swiftly to improve your life. To find out about our latest innovations, visit us at *https://laxiba.com* and register for our useletter.

Many improvements make this second edition the gold standard. Each contribution can help to make the book even better in the future. Thus, I am glad to learn about your experiences and your wishes! There are still grey areas, and regularly new foods enter the market that fit our tables well. To deal with the disease, it is important that you adapt your diet to the capacity of your enzyme workers. Therefore, we are interested in any food you are missing.

Would you like to take part in a coaching concerning the implementation of the diet or a workshop on stress management? We will have an offer that suits you. Visit us at *https://laxiba.com*. We look forward to getting to know you. Finally, I wish you prosperity, happiness and an improvement in your quality of life.

Your author,

Jan Stratbucker – *John@Laxiba.com*

3

FOOD TABLES

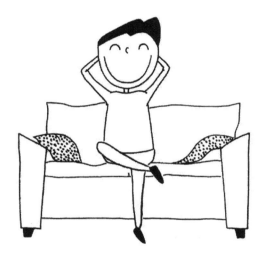

3.1   Introduction to the tables

In the following section, you will learn about the tolerable serving sizes for an intolerance towards fructose. The statements all relate to **one meal**, assuming **three meals** per day and that only eat one food containing fructose. The stated amounts expect you to consume three meals per day, one at roughly 7 am, 1 pm and 7 pm, i.e., each with about **six hours** in between. However, the times are mainly just a reference point just make sure to keep the gaps! If you read the book carefully, you have also learned that eating in between the big meals can have a positive effect on your health. For each food, you can find out how much you can tolerate both in a suitable unit as well as in gram. These statements make cooking as well as eating out easy.

The lists are ordered by category. Apple juice is listed under beverages-juices es, for example. The idea behind this is that you can easily find alternatives should your tolerated amount be small. At the end of the tables, you also find a food index, though, see page 219, which you can use if you are solely interested in finding out how much orange juice you can stomach.

The tables are set up in a manner that is easy to understand. Each page contains about 14 foods. In the tables, you find the category title in the first cell of each table. Below it, you can see the food names and next to them the tolerated amount explained by a proper unit or a smiley. Afterward, you find an explanation as well as the amount in gram. This procedure also concerns the B-factors for fructose—they indicate that the food is free of fructose and contains glucose. Due to this fact, you enhance your ability to eat foods containing fructose if you eat glucose containing foods with it. It is important to us that the data quality is excellent. All figures originate from an analysis conducted by the *University of Minnesota*. For the first time, the tables account for the interactions of fructose with glucose sorbitol to allow for a more reliable diet. In the following the symbols and units will be explained further.

3.1.1   Explanation of the symbols

Here you will find an explanation of the symbols. They show you at a glance how many units you can tolerate of the respective food. If you can see a smiley in the list, you will not find an amount. If the smiley looks sad, you should avoid the product if you have a fructose intolerance. If it smiles, you can enjoy it to your heart's content—if there is a big smile this also hold if you have a hereditary fructose intolerance.

Symbol	Meaning
	An average sized potion
	Slice(s)
	Piece(s)
	Hand(s) full
	Tablespoon(s)
	Bar
	Pinch
	Cup, 150 ml
	Glass, 200 ml
	Avoid the consumption. You can tolerate less than ¼ of the lowest amount due to the high fructose load of the food.
	Nearly free of fructose, hence, you can tolerate it unless you suffer from a hereditary fructose intolerance.

Symbol	Meaning

Free consumption as the food is free of fructose.

Glucose

The food is free of fructose. Moreover, it contains more glucose than fructose. Thus, the simultaneous intake of a portion measurement unit of the respective food can enable you to eat up to B-[number] times the amount of other fructose-containing foods. To be on the safe side, divide the [number] by two, as you partially absorb glucose by the mouth and sometimes the food you do not chew thoroughly. Hence, to profit from the glucose of another food, you should either mix both in advance or chew them together.

For example, for an ice cream you find "B ×3". For grapes, the tolerated amount is ¼. Hence, if you eat the grapes together with the ice cream, you can now consume ¼ plus ¼ ×3 and thus 1 unit. If you want to be on the safe side, divide the B-number by two, and you can consume about half a unit of grapes. Hint: If you can tolerate more than the standard amount, be aware that the B-multiplier works for the norm level only, i.e. calculate the additionally consumable amount by using the standard amount in the table.

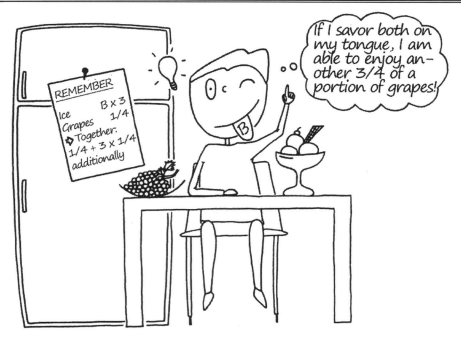

3.1.2   Explanation of the statements

Label	Meaning
Standard amount	In this column, you find the name of the unit or the meaning of the smiley. Behind it, in brackets, is stated how much gram one unit has followed by the tolerated amount per meal in total. For products that contain more glucose than fructose, you will also find the B-factor definition.
¼, ½, ¾, 1, 1¼, 1½, 1¾, 2, etc.	The tolerated amount of the respective unit, e.g., "cookie ½ piece" means you tolerate half a cookie of the type per meal, and "soup 1¾ portion" means one and three-fourths of a portion of the soup.
Avoid consumption.	Avoid the consumption of the food; it contains much fructose.
Avoid consumption!	Avoid the consumption of the food; it contains very much fructose.
Avoid consumption!!	Avoid the consumption of the food; it contains an extreme load fructose.

Note: Please always look at the ingredients as stated on the food packages as well. Especially, if the list does not mention a producer, the composition may vary. In addition, you should consider the weight of one unit in gram. The average portion sizes underlying the statements may be larger or smaller than you expect. For example, 30g of cereals may fill an entire bowl while you can eat 30g of a fruit in three bites.

3.1.3   Your personal sensitivity level

Level multiplier and fructose amount per meal by level

	Level	g	Table amount multiplier	Your level
Fructose g/meal	Standard	0.5	base	
	1	1	×2	
	2	2	×4	
	3	3	×6	

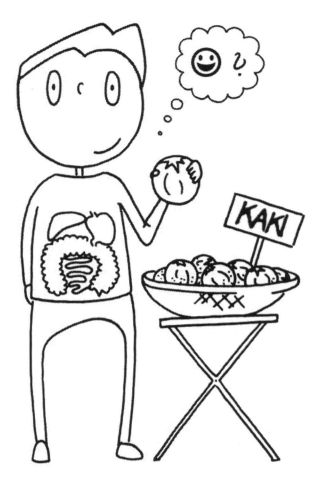

Check it with the Laxiba App!

1. Get it on the App Store or on Google Play and subscribe

2. Choose "Yes" or your tolerance level for your sensitivities

3. Find the answer with the text or category search option

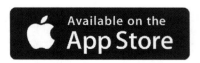
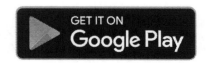

CATEGORY LIST-INDEX

3.2 Athletes

Athletes	FRUCTOSE		Standard amount
Clif Bar®, Chocolate Chip	B ×10	☺+	Free of fructose. Per Piece (68g) you eat with it, add B-no × F-limit.
Clif Bar®, Crunchy Peanut Butter	B ×10	☺+	Free of fructose. Per Piece (68g) you eat with it, add B-no × F-limit.
Clif Bar®, Oatmeal Raisin Walnut	B ×10	☺+	Free of fructose. Per Piece (68g) you eat with it, add B-no × F-limit.
Electrolyte replacement drink	B ×9¾	☺+	Free of fructose. Per Glass (200 mL) you drink with it, add B-no × F-limit.
Gatorade®, all flavors	B ×1¼	☺+	Free of fructose. Per Glass (200 mL) you drink with it, add B-no × F-limit.
Gatorade®, from dry mix, all flavors	B ×10	☺+	Free of fructose. Per Glass (200 mL) you drink with it, add B-no × F-limit.
Glaceau® Vitaminwater 10		☹	Avoid consumption.
Glaceau® Vitaminwater Energy		☹	Avoid consumption!
Glaceau® Vitaminwater Essential		☹	Avoid consumption!
Glaceau® Vitaminwater Focus		☹	Avoid consumption!
Glaceau® Vitaminwater Power-C		☹	Avoid consumption!
Glaceau® Vitaminwater Revive		☹	Avoid consumption!
High-protein Bar, generic	¾	🍰	Piece (65g); 49g in total.
Power Bar® 20g Protein Plus, Chocolate Crisp		☹	Avoid consumption!
Power Bar® 20g Protein Plus, Chocolate Peanut Butter		☹	Avoid consumption!!

Athletes	FRUCTOSE		Standard amount
Power Bar® 30g Protein Plus, Chocolate Brownie	B ×1½	☺+	Free of fructose. Per Piece (70g) you eat with it, add B-no × F-limit.
Power Bar® Harvest Energy®, Double Chocolate Crisp	B ×5¾	☺+	Free of fructose. Per Piece (65g) you eat with it, add B-no × F-limit.
Power Bar® Performance Energy®, Banana	¼		Piece (65g); 16g in total.
Power Bar® Performance Energy®, Chocolate	¼		Piece (65g); 16g in total.
Power Bar® Performance Energy®, Cookie Dough	¼		Piece (65g); 16g in total.
Power Bar® Performance Energy®, Mixed Berry Blast	¼		Piece (65g); 16g in total.
Power Bar® Performance Energy®, Vanilla Crisp	¼		Piece (65g); 16g in total.
Powerade®, all flavors	B ×1¼	☺+	Free of fructose. Per Glass (200 mL) you drink with it, add B-no × F-limit.

3.3 Beverages

3.3.1 Alcoholic

Alcoholic	FRUCTOSE		Standard amount
Ale		😀	Free of fructose.
Amaretto	B ×5	😊+	Free of fructose. Per Glass (200 mL) you drink with it, add B-no × F-limit.
Apple juice or cider, made from frozen		☹	Avoid consumption!
Apple juice or cider, un-sweetened		☹	Avoid consumption!
Applejack liquor		😃	Free of fructose.
Aquavit		😃	Free of fructose.
Beer		😀	Free of fructose.
Beer, low alcohol	B ×2¼	😊+	Free of fructose. Per Glass (200 mL) you drink with it, add B-no × F-limit.
Beer, low carb		😃	Free of fructose.
Beer, non alcoholic		😃	Free of fructose.
Black Russian		🙂	Nearly free of fructose, avoid at hereditary fructose intolerance.
Bloody Mary	1	🥛	Glass (200g); 200 ml in total.
Bourbon		😃	Free of fructose.
Brandy		😃	Free of fructose.
Brandy, flavored	B ×5	😊+	Free of fructose. Per Glass (200 mL) you drink with it, add B-no × F-limit.

Alcoholic	FRUCTOSE		Standard amount
Burgundy wine, red		😊	Free of fructose.
Burgundy wine, white		😊	Free of fructose.
Campari®	B ×5	😊+	Free of fructose. Per Glass (200 mL) you drink with it, add B-no × F-limit.
Cape Cod	B ×5	😊+	Free of fructose. Per Glass (200 mL) you drink with it, add B-no × F-limit.
Champagne punch	½	🥛	Glass (200g); 100 ml in total.
Champagne, white		😊	Free of fructose.
Chardonnay		😊	Free of fructose.
Club soda		😊	Free of fructose.
Cognac		😄	Free of fructose.
Cointreau®	B ×5	😊+	Free of fructose. Per Glass (200 mL) you drink with it, add B-no × F-limit.
Creme de Cocoa		😊	Nearly free of fructose, avoid at hereditary fructose intolerance.
Creme de menthe	B ×5	😊+	Free of fructose. Per Glass (200 mL) you drink with it, add B-no × F-limit.
Curacao	B ×5	😊+	Free of fructose. Per Glass (200 mL) you drink with it, add B-no × F-limit.
Daiquiri		😄	Free of fructose.
Eggnog, regular	B ×4¾	😊+	Free of fructose. Per Glass (200 mL) you drink with it, add B-no × F-limit.
Fruit punch, alcoholic	½	🥛	Glass (200g); 100 ml in total.

Alcoholic	FRUCTOSE		Standard amount
Gibson		😃	Free of fructose.
Gin		😃	Free of fructose.
Grand Marnier®	B ×5	😊+	Free of fructose. Per Glass (200 mL) you drink with it, add B-no × F-limit.
Grasshopper	B ×1½	😊+	Free of fructose. Per Glass (200 mL) you drink with it, add B-no × F-limit.
Harvey Wallbanger	62½	🥛	Glass (200g); 12500 ml in total.
Kamikaze	B ×1¾	😊+	Free of fructose. Per Glass (200 mL) you drink with it, add B-no × F-limit.
Kirsch	B ×5	😊+	Free of fructose. Per Glass (200 mL) you drink with it, add B-no × F-limit.
Light beer	B ×¼	😊+	Free of fructose. Per Glass (200 mL) you drink with it, add B-no × F-limit.
Liqueur, coffee flavored		😊	Nearly free of fructose, avoid at hereditary fructose intolerance.
Long Island iced tea	¾	🥛	Glass (200g); 150 ml in total.
Mai Tai	B ×½	😊+	Free of fructose. Per Glass (200 mL) you drink with it, add B-no × F-limit.
Malt liquor		😃	Free of fructose.
Manhattan	½	🥛	Glass (200g); 100 ml in total.
Margarita, frozen	B ×¼	😊+	Free of fructose. Per Glass (200 mL) you drink with it, add B-no × F-limit.
Martini®		😃	Free of fructose.
Merlot, red		😃	Free of fructose.

Alcoholic	FRUCTOSE	Standard amount
Merlot, white	¾	Glass (200g); 150 ml in total.
Mint Julep	☺	Free of fructose.
Mojito	☺	Free of fructose.
Muscatel	☹	Avoid consumption!
Non-alcoholic wine	2¼	Glass (200g); 450 ml in total.
Ouzo	B ×5	Free of fructose. Per Glass (200 mL) you drink with it, add B-no × F-limit.
Pina colada	B ×1¼	Free of fructose. Per Glass (200 mL) you drink with it, add B-no × F-limit.
Port wine	☹	Avoid consumption!
Riesling	☺	Free of fructose.
Rob Roy	¼	Glass (200g); 50 ml in total.
Rompope (eggnog with alcohol)	☺	Free of fructose.
Root beer	½	Glass (200g); 100 ml in total.
Rose wine, other types	¾	Glass (200g); 150 ml in total.
Rum	☺	Free of fructose.
Rum and cola	1	Glass (200g); 200 ml in total.
Rusty nail	B ×2	Free of fructose. Per Glass (200 mL) you drink with it, add B-no × F-limit.

Alcoholic	FRUCTOSE		Standard amount
Sake		😞	Avoid consumption!
Sambuca	B ×5	😊+	Free of fructose. Per Glass (200 mL) you drink with it, add B-no × F-limit.
Sangria	5½	🥛	Glass (200g); 1100 ml in total.
Schnapps, all flavors	B ×2½	😊+	Free of fructose. Per Glass (200 mL) you drink with it, add B-no × F-limit.
Scotch and soda		😊	Free of fructose.
Screwdriver	1	🥛	Glass (200g); 200 ml in total.
Seabreeze	B ×5¼	😊+	Free of fructose. Per Glass (200 mL) you drink with it, add B-no × F-limit.
Singapore sling	B ×¼	😊+	Free of fructose. Per Glass (200 mL) you drink with it, add B-no × F-limit.
Sloe gin	B ×5	😊+	Free of fructose. Per Glass (200 mL) you drink with it, add B-no × F-limit.
Sloe gin fizz	B ×¾	😊+	Free of fructose. Per Glass (200 mL) you drink with it, add B-no × F-limit.
Southern Comfort®		😊	Free of fructose.
Sylvaner		😊	Free of fructose.
Tequila		😊	Free of fructose.
Tequila sunrise	B ×¼	😊+	Free of fructose. Per Glass (200 mL) you drink with it, add B-no × F-limit.
Tokaji Wine		😞	Avoid consumption!
Tom Collins	22½	🥛	Glass (200g); 4500 ml in total.

Alcoholic	FRUCTOSE		Standard amount
Triple Sec	B ×5	😊	Free of fructose. Per Glass (200 mL) you drink with it, add B-no × F-limit.
Vodka		😊	Free of fructose.
Whiskey		😊	Free of fructose.
Whiskey sour	7¼	🥛	Glass (200g); 1450 ml in total.
White Russian		😊	Free of fructose.
Wine spritzer		😊	Free of fructose.

3.3.2 Hot beverages

Hot beverages	FRUCTOSE	Standard amount
Americano, decaf, without flavored syrup	😃	Free of fructose.
Americano, with flavored syrup	😃	Free of fructose.
Americano, without flavored syrup	😃	Free of fructose.
Brown sugar	😃	Free of fructose.
Cafe au lait, without flavored syrup	😃	Free of fructose.
Cafe latte, with flavored syrup	😃	Free of fructose.
Cafe latte, without flavored syrup	😃	Free of fructose.
Camomile tea	😃	Free of fructose.
Cappuccino, bottled or canned	😃	Free of fructose.
Cappuccino, decaf, with flavored syrup	😃	Free of fructose.
Cappuccino, decaf, without flavored syrup	😃	Free of fructose.
Chai tea	😃	Free of fructose.
Chicory coffee	🙂	Nearly free of fructose, avoid at hereditary fructose intolerance.
Coffee substitute, prepared	😃	Free of fructose.
Coffee, prepared from flavored mix, sugar free	😃	Free of fructose.

Hot beverages	FRUCTOSE	Standard amount
Dandelion tea	😊	Free of fructose.
Demitasse	😊	Free of fructose.
Dove® Promises, Milk Chocolate	😊	Free of fructose.
Earl Grey, strong	¾ 🥛	Glass (200g); 150 ml in total.
Espresso, without flavored syrup	😊	Free of fructose.
Evaporated milk, diluted, skim (fat free)	😊	Free of fructose.
Fennel tea	😊	Free of fructose.
Frappuccino®	😊	Free of fructose.
Frappuccino®, bottled or canned	😊	Free of fructose.
Frappuccino®, bottled or canned, light	😊	Free of fructose.
Green tea, strong	😊	Free of fructose.
Herbal tea	😊	Free of fructose.
Hershey's® Bliss Hot Drink White Chocolate, prepared	B ×½ 😊+	Free of fructose. Per Cup (150 mL) you drink with it, add B-no × F-limit.
Hot chocolate, homemade	25½ ☕	Cup (150g); 3825 ml in total.
Instant coffee mix, unprepared	4 ☕	Cup (150g); 600 ml in total.
Irish coffee with alcohol and whipped cream	😊	Free of fructose.

Hot beverages	FRUCTOSE		Standard amount
Jasmine tea		😊	Free of fructose.
Light cream		😊	Free of fructose.
Milk, lactose reduced Lactaid®, skim (fat free)	B ×7½	😊+	Free of fructose. Per Cup (150 mL) you drink with it, add B-no × F-limit.
Milk, lactose reduced Lactaid®, whole	B ×7½	😊+	Free of fructose. Per Cup (150 mL) you drink with it, add B-no × F-limit.
Milk, unprepared dry powder, nonfat, instant		😊	Free of fructose.
Mocha, without flavored syrup	B ×1¾	😊+	Free of fructose. Per Cup (150 mL) you drink with it, add B-no × F-limit.
Nestle® Hot Cocoa Dark Chocolate, prepared	B ×½	😊+	Free of fructose. Per Cup (150 mL) you drink with it, add B-no × F-limit.
Nestle® Hot Cocoa Rich Milk Chocolate, prepared		😊	Free of fructose.
Oolong tea		😊	Free of fructose.
Soy milk, chocolate, with sugar, not fortified		😊	Free of fructose.
Splenda®		😊	Free of fructose.
Starbucks® Hot Cocoa Double Chocolate, prepared	33¼	☕	Cup (150g); 4988 ml in total.
Starbucks® Hot Cocoa Salted Caramel, prepared	30¼	☕	Cup (150g); 4538 ml in total.
Sugar, white granulated		😊	Free of fructose.
Sweetened condensed milk		😊	Free of fructose.
Sweetened condensed milk, reduced fat		😊	Free of fructose.

Hot beverages	FRUCTOSE	Standard amount
Swiss Miss® Hot Cocoa Sensible Sweets Diet, sugar free, prepared	☺	Nearly free of fructose, avoid at hereditary fructose intolerance.
Whipped cream, aerosol	☺	Free of fructose.
Whipped cream, aerosol, fat free	B ×¼ ☺+	Free of fructose. Per Portion (5g) you eat with it, add B-no × F-limit.
White tea	☺	Free of fructose.
Zsweet®	☺	Free of fructose.

3.3.3 Juices

Juices	FRUCTOSE	Standard amount
Apple banana strawberry juice	☹	Avoid consumption.
Apple grape juice	☹	Avoid consumption!
Apricot nectar	B ×5 ☺+	Free of fructose. Per Glass (200 mL) you drink with it, add B-no × F-limit.
Arby's® orange juice	¾ 🥛	Glass (200g); 150 ml in total.
Black cherry juice	¼ 🥛	Glass (200g); 50 ml in total.
Black currant juice	B ×1½ ☺+	Free of fructose. Per Glass (200 mL) you drink with it, add B-no × F-limit.
Blackberry juice	¼ 🥛	Glass (200g); 50 ml in total.
Capri Sun®, all flavors	B ×1 ☺+	Free of fructose. Per Glass (200 mL) you drink with it, add B-no × F-limit.
Carrot juice	B ×1 ☺+	Free of fructose. Per Glass (200 mL) you drink with it, add B-no × F-limit.
Cranberry juice cocktail, with apple juice	☹	Avoid consumption.
Cranberry juice cocktail, with blueberry juice	☹	Avoid consumption.
Fruit drink or punch, ready to drink	B ×1 ☺+	Free of fructose. Per Glass (200 mL) you drink with it, add B-no × F-limit.
Grapefruit juice, unsweetened, white	B ×5 ☺+	Free of fructose. Per Glass (200 mL) you drink with it, add B-no × F-limit.
Kern's® Mango-Orange Nectar	☹	Avoid consumption.
Kern's® Strawberry Nectar	☹	Avoid consumption.

Juices	FRUCTOSE	Standard amount
Lemon juice, fresh	1¾	Glass (200g); 350 ml in total.
Libby's® Apricot Nectar		Avoid consumption.
Libby's® Banana Nectar		Avoid consumption.
Libby's® Juicy Juice®, Apple Grape		Avoid consumption!
Libby's® Juicy Juice®, Grape		Avoid consumption!
Libby's® Pear Nectar		Avoid consumption!
Lime juice, fresh	B ×¾	Free of fructose. Per Glass (200 mL) you drink with it, add B-no × F-limit.
Mango nectar	¾	Glass (200g); 150 ml in total.
Northland® Cranberry Juice, all flavors	B ×7¼	Free of fructose. Per Glass (200 mL) you drink with it, add B-no × F-limit.
Orange kiwi passion juice		Free of fructose.
Passion fruit juice	B ×3¾	Free of fructose. Per Glass (200 mL) you drink with it, add B-no × F-limit.
Peach juice	½	Glass (200g); 100 ml in total.
Pear juice		Avoid consumption!
Pineapple juice	B ×3¼	Free of fructose. Per Glass (200 mL) you drink with it, add B-no × F-limit.
Pineapple orange drink	¾	Glass (200g); 150 ml in total.
Pomegranate juice	1¼	Glass (200g); 250 ml in total.

Juices	FRUCTOSE	Standard amount
Raspberry juice	🙁	Avoid consumption!
Tomato juice	¾ 🥛	Glass (200g); 150 ml in total.
V-8® 100% A-C-E Vitamin Rich Vegetable Juice	¼ 🥛	Glass (200g); 50 ml in total.
Veryfine Cranberry Raspberry	🙁	Avoid consumption.

3.3.4   Other beverages

Other beverages	FRUCTOSE		Standard amount
7 UP®		☹	Avoid consumption!
Canfield's® Root Beer		☺	Free of fructose.
Canfield's® Root Beer, diet		☺	Free of fructose.
Cherry Coke®	½	🥛	Glass (200g); 100 ml in total.
Coke Zero®		☺	Free of fructose.
Coke®	½	🥛	Glass (200g); 100 ml in total.
Coke® with Lime	½	🥛	Glass (200g); 100 ml in total.
Diet 7 UP®		☺	Free of fructose.
Diet Coke®		☺	Free of fructose.
Diet Dr. Pepper®		☺	Free of fructose.
Diet Pepsi®, fountain		☺	Free of fructose.
Fanta Zero®, fruit flavors		☺	Free of fructose.
Fanta® Red		☹	Avoid consumption.
Fanta®, fruit flavors	8¼	🥛	Glass (200g); 1650 ml in total.
Ginger ale		☹	Avoid consumption!

Other beverages	FRUCTOSE		Standard amount
Lipton® Iced Tea Mix, with sugar, prepared		😊	Free of fructose.
Lipton® Instant 100% Tea, unsweetened, prepared		😊	Free of fructose.
Mineral Water		😊	Free of fructose.
Monster® Energy®	B ×17	😊+	Free of fructose. Per Glass (200 mL) you drink with it, add B-no × F-limit.
Monster® Khaos	B ×9½	😊+	Free of fructose. Per Portion (240g) you eat with it, add B-no × F-limit.
Mountain Dew®		😟	Avoid consumption.
Mountain Dew® Code Red		😟	Avoid consumption.
Nestea® 100% Tea, unsweetened, dry	B ×22	😊+	Free of fructose. Per Glass (200 mL) you drink with it, add B-no × F-limit.
Nestea® Iced Tea, Sugar Free, dry	B ×11	😊+	Free of fructose. Per Glass (200 mL) you drink with it, add B-no × F-limit.
Nestea® Iced Tea, Sugar Free, prepared		😊	Free of fructose.
Nestea® Iced Tea, sweetened with sugar, dry		😊	Free of fructose.
No Fear®	B ×6¼	😊+	Free of fructose. Per Glass (200 mL) you drink with it, add B-no × F-limit.
No Fear® Sugar Free		😊	Free of fructose.
Pepsi®	½	🥛	Glass (200g); 100 ml in total.
Pepsi® Max		😊	Free of fructose.
Pepsi® Twist	½	🥛	Glass (200g); 100 ml in total.

Other beverages	FRUCTOSE		Standard amount
Red Bull® Energy Drink	B ×7¾	😊+	Free of fructose. Per Glass (200 mL) you drink with it, add B-no × F-limit.
Red Bull® Energy Drink Sugar Free		😊	Free of fructose.
Rockstar Original®	B ×23	😊+	Free of fructose. Per Glass (200 mL) you drink with it, add B-no × F-limit.
Rockstar Original® Sugar Free		😊	Free of fructose.
Schweppes® Bitter Lemon		☹	Avoid consumption!
Spearmint tea		😊	Free of fructose.
Sprite®		☹	Avoid consumption!
Sprite® Zero		😊	Free of fructose.
Tap water		😊	Free of fructose.
Tonic water		☹	Avoid consumption!
Tonic water, diet		😊	Free of fructose.
Vanilla Coke®	½	🥛	Glass (200g); 100 ml in total.
Yerba® Mate tea		😊	Free of fructose.

3.4 Cold dishes

3.4.1 Bread

Bread	FRUCTOSE		Standard amount
Baguette		😊	Free of fructose.
Cracked wheat bread, with raisins	1¼	🤚	Slice (42g); 53g in total.
English muffin bread	38¼	🤚	Slice (42g); 1607g in total.
Focaccia bread		😊	Free of fructose.
French or Vienna roll		😊	Free of fructose.
GG® Scandinavian Bran Crispbread (Health Valley®)		🙂	Nearly free of fructose, avoid at hereditary fructose intolerance.
Gluten free bread		😊	Free of fructose.
Newman's Own® Organic Pretzels, Spelt	B ×½	🙂	Free of fructose. Per Slice (42g) you eat with it, add B-no × F-limit.
Potato bread		😊	Free of fructose.
Pumpernickel roll		😊	Free of fructose.
Rice bread		😊	Free of fructose.
Rye bread		😊	Free of fructose.
Rye roll		😊	Free of fructose.
Sourdough bread		😊	Free of fructose.

Bread	FRUCTOSE		Standard amount
Soy bread	5½		Slice (42g); 231g in total.
Toast, cinnamon and sugar, whole wheat bread	1½		Slice (42g); 63g in total.
Toast, wheat bread, with butter	1¾		Slice (42g); 74g in total.
Triticale bread	2½		Slice (42g); 105g in total.
White bread, store bought	1¼		Slice (42g); 53g in total.
White whole grain wheat bread	¾		Slice (42g); 32g in total.
Whole wheat bread, store bought	1¼		Slice (42g); 53g in total.

3.4.2 Cereals

Cereals	FRUCTOSE		Standard amount
All-Bran® Original (Kellogg's®)	B ×¼	😊 +	Free of fructose. Per Portion (30g) you eat with it, add B-no × F-limit.
Amaranth Flakes (Arrowhead Mills)	3		Portion (30g); 90g in total.
Cascadian Farm® Organic Granola Bar, Trail Mix Dark Chocolate Cranberry	B ×4¼	😊 +	Free of fructose. Per Piece (35g) you eat with it, add B-no × F-limit.
Cheerios® Snack Mix, all flavors	5		Portion (30g); 150g in total.
Chocolate Chex® (General Mills®)	¼	🥄	Tbsp. (15g); 4g in total.
Cinnamon toast crunch® (General Mills®)	¼		Portion (30g); 8g in total.
Cinnamon Toasters® (Malt-O-Meal®)	2		Portion (30g); 60g in total.
Cocoa Krispies® (Kellogg's®)		😄	Free of fructose.
Cocoa Puffs® (General Mills®)	B ×2	😊 +	Free of fructose. Per Portion (30g) you eat with it, add B-no × F-limit.
Corn Chex® (General Mills®)		😄	Free of fructose.
Corn Flakes (Kellogg's®)	B ×1½	😊 +	Free of fructose. Per Portion (30g) you eat with it, add B-no × F-limit.
Crunchy Nut Roasted Nut & Honey (Kellogg's®)	18¼		Portion (30g); 548g in total.
Essentials Oat Bran cereal (Quaker®)		😊	Free of fructose.
Evaporated milk, diluted, skim (fat free)		😊	Free of fructose.
Familia Swiss Muesli®, Original Recipe	¾		Portion (55g); 41g in total.

Cereals	FRUCTOSE		Standard amount
Fiber One Original® (General Mills®)	41½		Portion (30g); 1245g in total.
Fiber One® Nutty Clusters & Almonds (General Mills®)		☺	Free of fructose.
Froot Loops® (Kellogg's®)		☺	Free of fructose.
Frosted Flakes® (Kellogg's®)		☺	Free of fructose.
Frosted Flakes® Reduced Sugar (Kellogg's®)	B ×¼	☺+	Free of fructose. Per Portion (30g) you eat with it, add B-no × F-limit.
Frosted Mini-Wheats Big Bite® (Kellogg's®)	B ×¼	☺+	Free of fructose. Per Portion (55g) you eat with it, add B-no × F-limit.
GoLEAN® Crisp! Cereal, Cinnamon Crumble (Kashi®)	B ×1¼	☺+	Free of fructose. Per Portion (55g) you eat with it, add B-no × F-limit.
GoLEAN® Crunch! Cereal, Honey Almond Flax (Kashi®)	B ×1	☺+	Free of fructose. Per Portion (55g) you eat with it, add B-no × F-limit.
Health Valley® Multigrain Granola Bar, Chocolate Chip	B ×1	☺+	Free of fructose. Per Piece (29g) you eat with it, add B-no × F-limit.
Honey	½		Tbsp. (15g); 8g in total.
Honey Nut Chex® (General Mills®)		☺	Free of fructose.
Honey Smacks® (Kellogg's®)	B ×12	☺+	Free of fructose. Per Portion (30g) you eat with it, add B-no × F-limit.
Kashi® Chewy Granola Bar, Cherry Dark Chocolate	B ×1	☺+	Free of fructose. Per Piece (35g) you eat with it, add B-no × F-limit.
Maple syrup, pure	B ×¼	☺+	Free of fructose. Per Tbsp. (15g) you eat with it, add B-no × F-limit.
Milk, lactose reduced Lactaid®, skim (fat free) fortified with calcium or not	B ×10	☺+	Free of fructose. Per Glass (200 mL) you drink with it, add B-no × F-limit.

Cereals	FRUCTOSE		Standard amount
Mueslix® (Kellogg's®)	B ×¾	☺ +	Free of fructose. Per Portion (55g) you eat with it, add B-no × F-limit.
Rice Krispies® (Kellogg's®)		☺	Free of fructose.
Sorghum		☺	Free of fructose.
Special K® Blueberry cereal (Kellogg's®)	B ×½	☺ +	Free of fructose. Per Portion (30g) you eat with it, add B-no × F-limit.
Special K® Cinnamon Pecan cereal (Kellogg's®)		☺	Nearly free of fructose, avoid at hereditary fructose intolerance.
Special K® Original cereal (Kellogg's®)		☺	Free of fructose.
Special K® Red Berries cereal (Kellogg's®)		☺	Free of fructose.
Sprinkles Cookie Crisp® (General Mills®)	B ×¼	☺ +	Free of fructose. Per Portion (30g) you eat with it, add B-no × F-limit.
Sunbelt Bakery® Chewy Granola Bar, Banana Harvest	B ×¾	☺ +	Free of fructose. Per Piece (25g) you eat with it, add B-no × F-limit.
Sunbelt Bakery® Granola Bar, Blueberry Harvest	B ×¾	☺ +	Free of fructose. Per Piece (25g) you eat with it, add B-no × F-limit.
Sunbelt Bakery® Chewy Granola Bar, Golden Almond	B ×¾	☺ +	Free of fructose. Per Piece (28g) you eat with it, add B-no × F-limit.
Sunbelt Bakery® Granola Bar, Low Fat Oatmeal Raisin		☺	Free of fructose.
Sunbelt Bakery® Chewy Granola Bar, Oats & Honey	B ×¾	☺ +	Free of fructose. Per Piece (27g) you eat with it, add B-no × F-limit.
Sunbelt Bakery® Fudge Dipped Granola Bar, Coconut	B ×1¾	☺ +	Free of fructose. Per Piece (29g) you eat with it, add B-no × F-limit.
Weetabix® Organic Crispy Flakes & Fiber	B ×¾	☺ +	Free of fructose. Per Portion (55g) you eat with it, add B-no × F-limit.
Wheaties® (General Mills®)	83¼	🍳	Portion (30g); 2498g in total.

3.4.3   Cold cut

Cold cut	FRUCTOSE		Standard amount
Almond butter, salted		☺	Free of fructose.
Almond butter, unsalted		☺	Free of fructose.
Alpine Lace 25% Reduced Fat, Mozzarella		☺	Free of fructose.
American cheese, processed		☺	Free of fructose.
Blue cheese		☺	Free of fructose.
Bologna, beef ring	B ×5¾	☺+	Free of fructose. Per Portion (55g) you eat with it, add B-no × F-limit.
Bologna, combination of meats, light (reduced fat)	B ×½	☺+	Free of fructose. Per Portion (55g) you eat with it, add B-no × F-limit.
Brie cheese		☺	Free of fructose.
Butter, light, salted		☺	Free of fructose.
Butter, unsalted		☺	Free of fructose.
Camembert cheese		☺	Free of fructose.
Cheddar cheese, natural		☺	Free of fructose.
Cheese sauce, store bought		☺	Free of fructose.
Colby Jack cheese		☺	Free of fructose.
Cottage cheese, 1% fat, lactose reduced	B ×1¾	☺+	Free of fructose. Per Portion (110g) you eat with it, add B-no × F-limit.

Cold cut	FRUCTOSE		Standard amount
Cottage cheese, uncreamed dry curd		☺	Free of fructose.
Cream cheese spread		☺	Free of fructose.
Cream cheese, whipped, flavored		☺	Free of fructose.
Cream cheese, whipped, plain		☺	Free of fructose.
Edam cheese		☺	Free of fructose.
Fleischmann's® Move Over Butter Margarine, tub		☺	Free of fructose.
Goat cheese, hard		☺	Free of fructose.
Gorgonzola cheese		☺	Free of fructose.
Gouda cheese		☺	Free of fructose.
Honey	¼		Portion (21, 19g); 5g in total.
Hot dog, combination of meats, plain	B ×3	☺+	Free of fructose. Per Portion (55g) you eat with it, add B-no × F-limit.
Jam or preserves	B ×2¾	☺+	Free of fructose. Per Portion (20g) you eat with it, add B-no × F-limit.
Jam or preserves, reduced sugar	6¾		Portion (20g); 135g in total.
Jam or preserves, sugar free with aspartame	10½		Portion (17g); 179g in total.
Jam or preserves, sugar free with saccharin	2¼		Portion (14g); 32g in total.
Jam or preserves, sugar free with sucralose		☺	Free of fructose.

Cold cut	FRUCTOSE		Standard amount
Jam or preserves, without sugar or artificial sweetener	¼		Tbsp. (15g); 4g in total.
Kraft® Cheese Spread, Roka Blue			Free of fructose.
Limburger cheese			Free of fructose.
Maple syrup, pure	B ×¼		Free of fructose. Per Tbsp. (15g) you eat with it, add B-no × F-limit.
Margarine, diet, fat free			Free of fructose.
Margarine, tub, salted, sunflower oil			Free of fructose.
Marmalade, sugar free with aspartame	10½		Portion (17g); 179g in total.
Marmalade, sugar free with saccharin	2		Portion (16g); 32g in total.
Marmalade, sugar free with sucralose			Free of fructose.
Mascarpone			Free of fructose.
Mortadella	B ×¼		Free of fructose. Per Portion (55g) you eat with it, add B-no × F-limit.
Muenster cheese, natural			Free of fructose.
Nutella® (filbert spread)	40¾		Portion (37g); 1508g in total.
Roquefort cheese			Free of fructose.
Smart Balance® Light with Flax Oil Margarine, tub			Free of fructose.
Smart Balance® Margarine			Free of fructose.

Cold cut	FRUCTOSE		Standard amount
Soy Kaas Fat Free, all flavors	34½		Portion (30g); 1035g in total.
Swiss cheese, natural	B ×¼		Free of fructose. Per Portion (30g) you eat with it, add B-no × F-limit.
Swiss cheese, natural, low sodium	B ×¼		Free of fructose. Per Portion (30g) you eat with it, add B-no × F-limit.
Tilsit cheese			Free of fructose.

3.4.4 Dairy products

Dairy products	FRUCTOSE		Standard amount
Almond milk, vanilla or other flavors, unsweetened		😊	Free of fructose.
Breyers® Light! Boosts Immunity Yogurt, all flavors	21½	🍰	Piece (115g); 2473g in total.
Breyers® No Sugar Added Ice Cream, Vanilla		😊	Free of fructose.
Breyers® YoCrunch Light Nonfat Yogurt, with granola		😊	Free of fructose.
Cabot® Non Fat Yogurt, plain		😊	Free of fructose.
Cabot® Non Fat Yogurt, vanilla	22	🍰	Piece (150g); 3300g in total.
Chobani® Nonfat Greek Yogurt, Black Cherry		😊	Free of fructose.
Chobani® Nonfat Greek Yogurt, Lemon	B ×½	😊+	Free of fructose. Per Piece (150g) you eat with it, add B-no × F-limit.
Chobani® Nonfat Greek Yogurt, Peach	B ×1	😊+	Free of fructose. Per Piece (250g) you eat with it, add B-no × F-limit.
Chobani® Nonfat Greek Yogurt, Raspberry	B ×¾	😊+	Free of fructose. Per Piece (250g) you eat with it, add B-no × F-limit.
Chobani® Nonfat Greek Yogurt, Strawberry	B ×¾	😊+	Free of fructose. Per Piece (250g) you eat with it, add B-no × F-limit.
Chocolate pudding, store bought		😊	Free of fructose.
Chocolate pudding, store bought, sugar free		🙂	Nearly free of fructose, avoid at hereditary fructose intolerance.
Cottage cheese, uncreamed dry curd		😊	Free of fructose.

Dairy products	FRUCTOSE		Standard amount
Dannon® Activia® Light Yogurt, vanilla	¼		Piece (115g); 29g in total.
Dannon® Activia® Yogurt, plain			Free of fructose.
Dannon® Greek Yogurt, Honey	¼		Piece (150g); 38g in total.
Dannon® Greek Yogurt, Plain			Free of fructose.
Dannon® la Crème Yogurt, fruit flavors	¼		Piece (115g); 29g in total.
Evaporated milk, diluted, 2% fat (reduced fat)			Free of fructose.
Evaporated milk, diluted, skim (fat free)			Free of fructose.
Evaporated milk, diluted, whole			Free of fructose.
Feta cheese			Free of fructose.
Feta cheese, fat free			Free of fructose.
Fondue sauce	B ×¼		Free of fructose. Per Portion (53g) you eat with it, add B-no × F-limit.
GO Veggie!™ Rice Slices, all flavors			Free of fructose.
Greek yogurt, plain, nonfat,			Free of fructose.
Half and half			Free of fructose.
Kefir			Free of fructose.
Laughing Cow® Mini Babybel®, Cheddar			Free of fructose.

Dairy products	FRUCTOSE		Standard amount
Laughing Cow® Mini Ba-bybel®, Original		☺	Free of fructose.
Licuado, mango	¼	🥛	Glass (200g); 50 mL in total.
Light cream		☺	Free of fructose.
Milk, lactose reduced Lac-taid®, skim (fat free)	B ×10	☺+	Free of fructose. Per Glass (200 mL) you drink with it, add B-no × F-limit.
Milk, lactose reduced Lac-taid®, whole	B ×10	☺+	Free of fructose. Per Glass (200 mL) you drink with it, add B-no × F-limit.
Milk, lactose reduced, skim (fat free), calcium Lactaid®	B ×10	☺+	Free of fructose. Per Glass (200 mL) you drink with it, add B-no × F-limit.
Mozzarella cheese, fat free		☺	Free of fructose.
Mozzarella cheese, whole milk		☺	Free of fructose.
Oat milk		☺	Nearly free of fructose, avoid at hered-itary fructose intolerance.
Parmesan cheese, dry (grated)		☺	Free of fructose.
Parmesan cheese, dry (grated), nonfat		☺	Free of fructose.
Pudding mix, other flavors, cooked type		☺	Free of fructose.
Rice milk, plain or original, unsweetened, enriched, ready	B ×¼	☺+	Free of fructose. Per Glass (200 mL) you drink with it, add B-no × F-limit.
Rice pudding (arroz con leche), coconut, raisins	4	🍰	Piece (200g); 800g in total.
Rice pudding (arroz con leche), plain	B ×½	☺+	Free of fructose. Per Piece (200g) you eat with it, add B-no × F-limit.
Rice pudding (arroz con leche), raisins	4	🍰	Piece (200g); 800g in total.

Dairy products	FRUCTOSE	Standard amount
Ricotta cheese, part skim milk	😊	Free of fructose.
Slim-Fast® Easy to Digest, Vanilla, ready-to-drink can	😊	Free of fructose.
Sour cream	😊	Free of fructose.
Soy milk, plain or original, artificial sweetener, ready	3 🥛	Glass (200g); 600 mL in total.
Soy milk, vanilla or other flavors, sugar, fat free, ready	B ×¾ 😊+	Free of fructose. Per Glass (200 mL) you drink with it, add B-no × F-limit.
Stonyfield® Oikos Greek Yogurt, Blueberry	B ×1 😊+	Free of fructose. Per Piece (250g) you eat with it, add B-no × F-limit.
Stonyfield® Oikos Greek Yogurt, Caramel	B ×½ 😊+	Free of fructose. Per Piece (100g) you eat with it, add B-no × F-limit.
Stonyfield® Oikos Greek Yogurt, Chocolate	66½ 🍰	Piece (150g); 9975g in total.
Stonyfield® Oikos Greek Yogurt, Strawberry	3 🍰	Piece (250g); 750g in total.
Strawberry milk, plain, prepared	😊	Free of fructose.
Sweetened condensed milk	😊	Free of fructose.
Sweetened condensed milk, reduced fat	😊	Free of fructose.
Tofu, raw (not silken), cooked, low fat	1½ 🍳	Portion (85g); 128g in total.
Whipped cream, aerosol	😊	Free of fructose.
Whipped cream, aerosol, chocolate	😊	Free of fructose.
Whipped cream, aerosol, fat free	B ×¼ 😊+	Free of fructose. Per Portion (5g) you eat with it, add B-no × F-limit.

Dairy products	FRUCTOSE		Standard amount
Yogurt, chocolate or coffee flavors, nonfat, aspartame		☺	Free of fructose.
Yogurt, chocolate or coffee flavors, whole milk, sucralose	40	🍰	Piece (250g); 10000g in total.
Yogurt, fruited, whole milk	¾	🥄	Tbsp. (15g); 11g in total.

3.4.5 Nuts and snacks

Nuts and snacks	FRUCTOSE		Standard amount
Almonds, raw		☺	Free of fructose.
Baby food, zwieback		☺	Free of fructose.
Brazil nuts, unsalted		☺	Free of fructose.
Caramel or sugar coated popcorn, store bought	B ×1	☺+	Free of fructose. Per Hand (21g) you eat with it, add B-no × F-limit.
Cashews, raw		☺	Free of fructose.
Cheese cracker		☺	Nearly free of fructose, avoid at hereditary fructose intolerance.
Chestnuts, roasted	83¼	🍳	Portion (30g); 2498g in total.
Chia seeds		☺	Free of fructose.
Coconut cream (liquid from grated meat)	20¾	🥥	Hand (30g); 623g in total.
Coconut milk, fresh (liquid from grated meat, water added)	B ×1	☺+	Free of fructose. Per Glass (200 mL) you drink with it, add B-no × F-limit.
Coconut, dried, shredded or flaked, unsweetened	B ×¾	☺+	Free of fructose. Per Hand (30g) you eat with it, add B-no × F-limit.
Coconut, fresh	B ×¼	☺+	Free of fructose. Per Portion (15g) you eat with it, add B-no × F-limit.
Doritos® Tortilla Chips, Nacho Cheese		☺	Free of fructose.
Filberts, raw		☺	Free of fructose.
Flax seeds, not fortified		☺	Free of fructose.

Nuts and snacks	FRUCTOSE	Standard amount
Ginko nuts, dried	☺	Nearly free of fructose, avoid at hereditary fructose intolerance.
Hickorynuts	☺	Free of fructose.
Lay's® Potato Chips, Classic	37¾	Hand (21g); 793g in total.
Lay's® Potato Chips, Salt & Vinegar	37¾	Hand (21g); 793g in total.
Lay's® Potato Chips, Sour Cream & Onion	37¾	Hand (21g); 793g in total.
Lay's® Stax Potato Crisps, Cheddar	37¾	Hand (21g); 793g in total.
Lay's® Stax Potato Crisps, Hot 'n Spicy Barbecue	49½	Hand (21g); 1040g in total.
Macadamia nuts, raw	☺	Free of fructose.
Melba Toast®, Classic (Old London®)	B ×¼ ☺+	Free of fructose. Per Portion (15g) you eat with it, add B-no × F-limit.
Old Dutch® Crunch Curls	☺	Free of fructose.
Peanut butter, unsalted	B ×¼ ☺+	Free of fructose. Per Portion (32g) you eat with it, add B-no × F-limit.
Peanuts, dry roasted, salted	☺	Free of fructose.
Pine nuts, pignolias	☺	Free of fructose.
Pistachio nuts, raw	☺	Free of fructose.
Poore Brothers® Potato Chips, Salt & Cracked Pepper	49½	Hand (21g); 1040g in total.
Potato chips, salted	37¾	Hand (21g); 793g in total.

Nuts and snacks	FRUCTOSE	Standard amount
Potato sticks	☺	Free of fructose.
Pretzels, hard, unsalted, sticks	☺	Free of fructose.
Pringles® Light Fat Free Potato Crisps, Barbecue	34	Hand (21g); 714g in total.
Pringles® Potato Crisps, Loaded Baked Potato	37¾	Hand (21g); 793g in total.
Pringles® Potato Crisps, Original	68	Hand (21g); 1428g in total.
Pringles® Potato Crisps, Salt & Vinegar	37¾	Hand (21g); 793g in total.
Pumpkin or squash seeds, shelled, unsalted	☺	Free of fructose.
Rice cake	☺	Free of fructose.
Ritz Cracker (Nabisco®)	☺	Free of fructose.
Sesame sticks	☺	Free of fructose.
Soy chips	7½	Hand (21g); 158g in total.
Sunflower seeds, raw	☺	Free of fructose.
Taco John's® nachos	☺	Free of fructose.
Tortilla, white, store bought, fried	☺	Free of fructose.
Walnuts	☺	Nearly free of fructose, avoid at hereditary fructose intolerance.
Wise Onion Flavored Rings	☺	Free of fructose.

3.4.6　Sweet pastries

Sweet pastries	FRUCTOSE	Standard amount
Almond cookies	☺	Free of fructose.
Apple cake, glazed	¾	Piece (45g); 34g in total.
Apple strudel	¼	Piece (64g); 16g in total.
Archway® Ginger Snaps	28½	Portion (30g); 855g in total.
Archway® Oatmeal Raisin Cookies	☺	Free of fructose.
Archway® Peanut Butter Cookies	2	Piece (34g); 68g in total.
Biscotti, chocolate, nuts	☺	Free of fructose.
Brownie, chocolate, fat free	66¾	Piece (44g); 2937g in total.
Butter cracker	☺	Free of fructose.
Carrot cake, glazed, home-made	B ×¼	Free of fructose. Per Piece (27.72g) you eat with it, add B-no × F-limit.
Cheesecake, plain or flavored, graham cracker crust, home-made	B ×½	Free of fructose. Per Piece (220g) you eat with it, add B-no × F-limit.
Cherry pie, bottom crust only	B ×1½	Free of fructose. Per Piece (122g) you eat with it, add B-no × F-limit.
Chips Ahoy!® Chewy Gooey Caramel Cookies (Nabisco®)	½	Piece (15.5g); 8g in total.
Chocolate cake, glazed, store bought	B ×½	Free of fructose. Per Piece (29g) you eat with it, add B-no × F-limit.

Sweet pastries	FRUCTOSE		Standard amount
Chocolate chip cookies, store bought		☺	Free of fructose.
Chocolate cookies, iced, store bought		☺	Free of fructose.
Chocolate sandwich cookies, double filling		☺	Free of fructose.
Chocolate sandwich cookies, sugar free		☺	Free of fructose.
Cinnamon crispas (fried flour tortilla, cinnamon, sugar)		☺	Free of fructose.
Crepe, plain		☺	Free of fructose.
Croissant, chocolate	B ×1	☺+	Free of fructose. Per Piece (69g) you eat with it, add B-no × F-limit.
Croissant, fruit	B ×2½	☺+	Free of fructose. Per Piece (74g) you eat with it, add B-no × F-limit.
Danish pastry, frosted or glazed, with cheese filling		☺	Free of fructose.
Dare Breaktime Ginger Cookies		☺	Nearly free of fructose, avoid at hereditary fructose intolerance.
Dare® Lemon Crème Cookies		☺	Free of fructose.
Doughnut, raised, glazed, coconut topping		☺	Free of fructose.
Doughnut, raised, glazed, plain		☺	Free of fructose.
Doughnut, raised, sugared		☺	Free of fructose.
EGG® bread roll		☺	Free of fructose.
Elephant ear (crispy)		☺	Free of fructose.

Sweet pastries	FRUCTOSE		Standard amount
English muffin, whole wheat, with raisins	2		Piece (66g); 132g in total.
French toast, homemade, French bread	B ×½		Free of fructose. Per Piece (131g) you eat with it, add B-no × F-limit.
Frozen custard, chocolate or coffee flavors	B ×2¼		Free of fructose. Per Portion (87.5g) you eat with it, add B-no × F-limit.
German chocolate cake, glazed, homemade	B ×½		Free of fructose. Per Piece (29g) you eat with it, add B-no × F-limit.
Girl Scout® Lemonades			Free of fructose.
Girl Scout® Peanut Butter Patties			Free of fructose.
Girl Scout® Samoas®			Free of fructose.
Girl Scout® Shortbread®			Free of fructose.
Girl Scout® Thin Mints			Nearly free of fructose, avoid at hereditary fructose intolerance.
Halvah	B ×1½		Free of fructose. Per Portion (40g) you eat with it, add B-no × F-limit.
Lebkuchen (German ginger bread)	5¼		Piece (32.4g); 170g in total.
Little Debbie® Coffee Cake, Apple Streusel	¾		Piece (52g); 39g in total.
Little Debbie® Fudge Brownies with Walnuts	B ×4¼		Free of fructose. Per Piece (30.5g) you eat with it, add B-no × F-limit.
Long John / Bismarck, glazed, cream or custard & nuts			Free of fructose.
Molasses cookies, store bought			Nearly free of fructose, avoid at hereditary fructose intolerance.
Muffins, banana	B ×¼		Free of fructose. Per Piece (113g) you eat with it, add B-no × F-limit.

Sweet pastries	FRUCTOSE		Standard amount
Muffins, blueberry, store bought	25½		Piece (113g); 2882g in total.
Muffins, carrot, homemade, with nuts			Free of fructose.
Muffins, oat bran or oatmeal, store bought	B ×¼		Free of fructose. Per Piece (113g) you eat with it, add B-no × F-limit.
Muffins, pumpkin, store bought	B ×¼		Free of fructose. Per Piece (113g) you eat with it, add B-no × F-limit.
Murray® Sugar Free Oatmeal Cookies			Free of fructose.
Murray® Sugar Free Short-bread			Free of fructose.
Nabisco® 100 Calorie Packs, Honey Maid Cinnamon Roll			Free of fructose.
Nilla Wafers® (Nabisco®)			Free of fructose.
Nutter Butter® Cookies (Nabisco®)			Free of fructose.
Oatmeal cookies, store bought			Free of fructose.
Oreo® Brownie Cookies (Nabisco®)	¼		Piece (42.5g); 11g in total.
Oreo® Cookies (Nabisco®)			Free of fructose.
Oreo® Cookies, Sugar Free (Nabisco®)			Free of fructose.
Pancake, buckwheat, from mix, add water only			Free of fructose.
Pancake, whole wheat, home-made			Free of fructose.
Peach pie, bottom crust only	2¾		Piece (122g); 336g in total.

Sweet pastries	FRUCTOSE	Standard amount
Pepperidge Farm® Sweet & Simple, Soft Sugar Cookies	☹	Avoid consumption.
Pepperidge Farm® Turnover, Apple	½	Piece (89g); 45g in total.
Pillsbury® Big White Chunk Macadamia Nut Cookies	☺	Nearly free of fructose, avoid at hereditary fructose intolerance.
Pillsbury® Cinnamon Roll with Icing, all flavors	B ×8¼ ☺+	Free of fructose. Per Piece (44g) you eat with it, add B-no × F-limit.
Popcorn, store bought (prepopped), "buttered"	☺	Free of fructose.
Rhubarb pie, bottom crust only	☺	Free of fructose.
Sandwich cookies, vanilla	☺	Free of fructose.
Sticky bun	B ×¾ ☺+	Free of fructose. Per Piece (71g) you eat with it, add B-no × F-limit.
Strawberry pie, bottom crust only	1¼	Piece (122g); 153g in total.
Sugar cookies, iced, store bought	☺	Free of fructose.
Sweet potato bread	☺	Free of fructose.
Tiramisu	☺	Free of fructose.
Twix®	B ×1½ ☺+	Free of fructose. Per Piece (51g) you eat with it, add B-no × F-limit.
Waffles, bran	B ×¼ ☺+	Free of fructose. Per Piece (95g) you eat with it, add B-no × F-limit.
Waffles, whole wheat, from mix, add milk, fat and egg	B ×¼ ☺+	Free of fructose. Per Piece (95g) you eat with it, add B-no × F-limit.
Windmill cookies	☺	Nearly free of fructose, avoid at hereditary fructose intolerance.

3.4.7 Sweets

Sweets	FRUCTOSE	Standard amount
3 Musketeers®	B ×3¾ ☺+	Free of fructose. Per Piece (60.4g) you eat with it, add B-no × F-limit.
After Eight® Thin Chocolate Mints	☺	Free of fructose.
Almond paste (Marzipan)	☺	Nearly free of fructose, avoid at hereditary fructose intolerance.
Almonds, honey roasted	1¾	Hand (30g); 53g in total.
Breath mint, regular	B ×¼ ☺+	Free of fructose. Per Portion (2g) you eat with it, add B-no × F-limit.
Breath mint, sugar free	☺	Free of fructose.
Brown sugar	☺	Free of fructose.
Buttermels® (Switzer's®)	B ×½ ☺+	Free of fructose. Per Piece (6.9g) you eat with it, add B-no × F-limit.
Candy necklace	B ×3¼ ☺+	Free of fructose. Per Piece (21g) you eat with it, add B-no × F-limit.
Chewing gum	☺	Free of fructose.
Chewing gum, sugar free	☺	Free of fructose.
Chocolate truffles	☺	Free of fructose.
Classic Fruit Chocolates (Liberty Orchards®)	B ×¼ ☺+	Free of fructose. Per Piece (15g) you eat with it, add B-no × F-limit.
Coconut Bars, nuts	☺	Free of fructose.
Dark chocolate Bar 45%-59% cacao	☺	Free of fructose.

Sweets	FRUCTOSE		Standard amount
Dark chocolate Bar 60%-69% cacao		☺	Free of fructose.
Dark chocolate Bar 70%-85% cacao		☺	Free of fructose.
Dark chocolate Bar, sugar free	17	🍰	Piece (12g); 204g in total.
Dark Fruit Chocolates (Liberty Orchards®)	B ×¼	☺+	Free of fructose. Per Piece (15g) you eat with it, add B-no × F-limit.
Dark Fruit Chocolates, Sugar Free (Liberty Orchards®)		☺	Free of fructose.
Fifty 50® Sugar Free Low Glycemic Butterscotch Hard Candy		☺	Free of fructose.
French Burnt Peanuts	B ×1¾	☺+	Free of fructose. Per Hand (30g) you eat with it, add B-no × F-limit.
Gelatin (jello) powder, flavored, sugar free		☺	Free of fructose.
Gelatin (jello) powder, plain		☺	Free of fructose.
Gum drops	B ×2¼	☺+	Free of fructose. Per Hand (30g) you eat with it, add B-no × F-limit.
Gum drops, sugar free		☺	Free of fructose.
Gummi bears	B ×3½	☺+	Free of fructose. Per Hand (30g) you eat with it, add B-no × F-limit.
Gummi bears, sugar free		☺	Free of fructose.
Gummi dinosaurs	B ×3½	☺+	Free of fructose. Per Hand (30g) you eat with it, add B-no × F-limit.
Gummi dinosaurs, sugar free		☺	Free of fructose.
Gummi worms	B ×3½	☺+	Free of fructose. Per Hand (30g) you eat with it, add B-no × F-limit.

Sweets	FRUCTOSE	Standard amount
Gummi worms, sugar free	🙂	Free of fructose.
Hard candy	B ×¾ 🙂+	Free of fructose. Per Piece (6g) you eat with it, add B-no × F-limit.
Hard candy, sugar free	🙂	Free of fructose.
Hershey's® Caramel Filled Chocolates Sugar Free	🙂	Free of fructose.
Hershey's® Milk Chocolate Bar	🙂	Free of fructose.
Jelly beans®	B ×9¾ 🙂+	Free of fructose. Per Hand (30g) you eat with it, add B-no × F-limit.
Jelly beans®, sugar free	🙂	Free of fructose.
Jujyfruits®	B ×12 🙂+	Free of fructose. Per Hand (30g) you eat with it, add B-no × F-limit.
Kashi® Layered Granola Bar, Pumpkin Pecan	B ×1½ 🙂+	Free of fructose. Per Piece (40g) you eat with it, add B-no × F-limit.
Kit Kat®	🙂	Free of fructose.
Kit Kat® White	🙂	Free of fructose.
Licorice	B ×1½ 🙂+	Free of fructose. Per Piece (11g) you eat with it, add B-no × F-limit.
Little Debbie® Nutty Bars	B ×13 🙂+	Free of fructose. Per Piece (28.5g) you eat with it, add B-no × F-limit.
M & M's® Peanut	🙂	Free of fructose.
Mamba® Fruit Chews	B ×22 🙂+	Free of fructose. Per Portion (40g) you eat with it, add B-no × F-limit.
Mamba® Sour Fruit Chews	B ×17 🙂+	Free of fructose. Per Portion (40g) you eat with it, add B-no × F-limit.

Sweets	FRUCTOSE		Standard amount
Marshmallow	B ×4½	☺+	Free of fructose. Per Portion (30g) you eat with it, add B-no × F-limit.
Mentos®		☺	Free of fructose.
Milk chocolate Bar, cereal		☺	Free of fructose.
Milk chocolate Bar, cereal, sugar free	40	🍰	Piece (12g); 480g in total.
Milk chocolate Bar, sugar free	40	🍰	Piece (12g); 480g in total.
Milk Chocolate covered raisins	B ×¼	☺+	Free of fructose. Per Hand (30g) you eat with it, add B-no × F-limit.
Milk Maid® Caramels (Brach's®)	B ×5¾	☺+	Free of fructose. Per Piece (40g) you eat with it, add B-no × F-limit.
Molasses, dark	3¾	🥄	Tbsp. (15g); 56g in total.
Nestle® Nesquik®, chocolate flavors, unprepared dry	1½	🥛	Glass (200g); 300 mL in total.
Nougat	B ×18	☺+	Free of fructose. Per Bar (125g) you eat with it, add B-no × F-limit.
Pecan praline	B ×1¼	☺+	Free of fructose. Per Piece (55g) you eat with it, add B-no × F-limit.
Riesen®	B ×2¾	☺+	Free of fructose. Per Piece (9g) you eat with it, add B-no × F-limit.
Smarties®	B ×55	☺+	Free of fructose. Per Hand (30g) you eat with it, add B-no × F-limit.
Snickers®	B ×7	☺+	Free of fructose. Per Piece (58.7g) you eat with it, add B-no × F-limit.
Snickers®, Almond	B ×8¾	☺+	Free of fructose. Per Piece (49.9g) you eat with it, add B-no × F-limit.
Splenda®		☺	Free of fructose.

Sweets	FRUCTOSE		Standard amount
Starburst®, Original	B ×½	☺ +	Free of fructose. Per Piece (5g) you eat with it, add B-no × F-limit.
Suckers®, sugar free		☺	Free of fructose.
Sugar, white granulated		☺	Free of fructose.
Taffy	B ×4¼	☺ +	Free of fructose. Per Piece (8.6g) you eat with it, add B-no × F-limit.
Tic Tacs®		☺	Free of fructose.
Toblerone® Swiss Dark Chocolate with Honey & Almond Nougat		☺	Free of fructose.
Toblerone® Swiss Milk Chocolate with Honey & Almond Nougat		☺	Free of fructose.
Toblerone® Swiss White Confection with Honey & Almond Nougat		☺	Free of fructose.
Toffee		☺	Free of fructose.
Toffifay®	B ×¼	☺ +	Free of fructose. Per Piece (8.2g) you eat with it, add B-no × F-limit.
Tootsie Pops®	B ×2½	☺ +	Free of fructose. Per Piece (17g) you eat with it, add B-no × F-limit.
Werther's® Original Caramel Coffee Hard Candies	B ×½	☺ +	Free of fructose. Per Piece (4g) you eat with it, add B-no × F-limit.
White chocolate Bar		☺	Free of fructose.
Wild 'n Fruity Gummi Bears (Brach's®)	B ×3½	☺ +	Free of fructose. Per Hand (30g) you eat with it, add B-no × F-limit.
Zsweet®		☺	Free of fructose.

3.5 Warm dishes

3.5.1 Meals

Meals	FRUCTOSE		Standard amount
Arby's® macaroni and cheese		☺	Free of fructose.
Asian noodle bowl, vegetables only	B ×1	☺+	Free of fructose. Per Portion (200g) you eat with it, add B-no × F-limit.
Baby food, Gerber Graduates® Organic Pasta Pick-Ups Three Cheese Ravioli		☺	Free of fructose.
Beef with noodles soup, condensed		☺	Free of fructose.
Boston Market® macaroni and cheese		☺	Free of fructose.
Butternut squash soup		☺	Free of fructose.
Calzone, cheese		☺	Free of fructose.
Casserole (hot dish), pasta with turkey, gravy base, vegetables except dark green, & cheese		☺	Free of fructose.
Casserole (hot dish), rice with beef, tomato base, vegetables except dark green, & cheese	B ×1	☺+	Free of fructose. Per Portion (244g) you eat with it, add B-no × F-limit.
Chicken and dumplings soup, condensed		☺	Free of fructose.
Chicken noodle soup with vegetables, ready-to-serve can		☺	Free of fructose.
Chicken wonton soup, prepared from condensed can		☺	Free of fructose.
Chili with beans, beef, canned	87½	🥄	Tbsp. (15g); 1313g in total.

Meals	FRUCTOSE	Standard amount
Chop suey, chicken, no noodles	😊	Free of fructose.
Chop suey, tofu, no noodles	😊	Free of fructose.
Cream of asparagus soup, prepared condensed can	😊	Nearly free of fructose, avoid at hereditary fructose intolerance.
Cream of broccoli soup, condensed	😊	Free of fructose.
Cream of celery soup, home-made	😊	Free of fructose.
Cream of chicken soup, condensed	😊	Nearly free of fructose, avoid at hereditary fructose intolerance.
Cream of mushroom soup, prepared condensed can	😊	Nearly free of fructose, avoid at hereditary fructose intolerance.
Cream of potato soup mix, dry	😊	Free of fructose.
Cream of spinach soup mix, dry	B ×¼ 😊+	Free of fructose. Per Portion (17g) you eat with it, add B-no × F-limit.
Dairy Queen® Foot Long Hot Dog	B ×1¾ 😊+	Free of fructose. Per Piece (199g) you eat with it, add B-no × F-limit.
Fettuccini Alfredo®, no meat, vegetables except dark green	😊	Free of fructose.
Fettuccini Alfredo®, no meat, carrots / dark green vegetables	😊	Free of fructose.
Fruit sauce, jelly-based	B ×5¼ 😊+	Free of fructose. Per Portion (40g) you eat with it, add B-no × F-limit.
German style potato salad, bacon and vinegar dressing	B ×¼ 😊+	Free of fructose. Per Portion (140g) you eat with it, add B-no × F-limit.
Green pea soup, prepared from condensed can	😊	Free of fructose.
Hardee's® Loaded Omelet Biscuit	B ×9¼ 😊+	Free of fructose. Per Piece (158g) you eat with it, add B-no × F-limit.

Meals	FRUCTOSE		Standard amount
Lasagna, homemade, beef	B ×¼	☺ +	Free of fructose. Per Portion (140g) you eat with it, add B-no × F-limit.
Lasagna, homemade, cheese, no vegetables	6		Portion (140g); 840g in total.
Lasagna, homemade, spinach, no meat	5½		Portion (140g); 770g in total.
Lentil soup, condensed		☺	Free of fructose.
Lyonnaise (potatoes and onions)		☺	Free of fructose.
Macaroni or pasta salad, with meat, egg, mayo dressing	B ×½	☺ +	Free of fructose. Per Portion (140g) you eat with it, add B-no × F-limit.
Meat ravioli, with tomato sauce	B ×½	☺ +	Free of fructose. Per Portion (250g) you eat with it, add B-no × F-limit.
Minestrone soup, condensed		☺	Free of fructose.
Minestrone soup, homemade		☺	Free of fructose.
Noodle soup mix, dry	B ×¼	☺ +	Free of fructose. Per Portion (16g) you eat with it, add B-no × F-limit.
Omelet, made with bacon	B ×1¾	☺ +	Free of fructose. Per Portion (110g) you eat with it, add B-no × F-limit.
Omelet, made with sausage, potatoes, onions, cheese	B ×1	☺ +	Free of fructose. Per Portion (110g) you eat with it, add B-no × F-limit.
Pad Thai, without meat		☺	Free of fructose.
Paella	2		Portion (240g); 480g in total.
Panda Express® Orange Chicken	¼		Portion (140g); 35g in total.
Pasta salad with vegetables, Italian dressing	2½		Portion (140g); 350g in total.

Meals	FRUCTOSE		Standard amount
Pho soup (Vietnamese noodle soup)		☺	Free of fructose.
Pizza Hut® cheese bread stick	B ×¼	☺+	Free of fructose. Per Piece (56g) you eat with it, add B-no × F-limit.
Pizza Hut® Pepperoni Lover's pizza, stuffed crust		☺	Free of fructose.
Pizza Hut® Personal Pan, supreme		☺	Free of fructose.
Pizza, homemade or restaurant, cheese, thin crust	B ×¾	☺+	Free of fructose. Per Piece (209g) you eat with it, add B-no × F-limit.
Potato salad, with egg, mayo dressing	B ×½	☺+	Free of fructose. Per Portion (140g) you eat with it, add B-no × F-limit.
Potato soup with broccoli and cheese		☺	Free of fructose.
Ratatouille		☺	Free of fructose.
Red beans and rice soup mix, dry	¼	🍜	Portion (51.03g); 13g in total.
Scrambled egg, made with bacon	B ×1¾	☺+	Free of fructose. Per Portion (110g) you eat with it, add B-no × F-limit.
Sesame chicken		☺	Free of fructose.
Soup base	54½	🥄	Tbsp. (15g); 818g in total.
Spaghetti, with carbonara sauce	B ×¾	☺+	Free of fructose. Per Portion (201g) you eat with it, add B-no × F-limit.
Spinach ravioli, with tomato sauce	B ×¼	☺+	Free of fructose. Per Portion (250g) you eat with it, add B-no × F-limit.
Spring roll	10½	🍜	Portion (140g); 1470g in total.
Squash or pumpkin ravioli, with cream sauce	B ×¼	☺+	Free of fructose. Per Portion (250g) you eat with it, add B-no × F-limit.

Meals	FRUCTOSE		Standard amount
Stewed green peas with sofrito		😊	Free of fructose.
Sushi, with fish	16	🍽	Portion (140g); 2240g in total.
Sushi, with fish and vegetables in seaweed		😊	Free of fructose.
Sushi, with vegetables in seaweed		😊	Free of fructose.
Swedish Meatballs		😊	Free of fructose.
Sweet and sour chicken	2½	🥄	Tbsp. (15g); 38g in total.
Taco Bell® 7-Layer Burrito		😊	Free of fructose.
Taco Bell® Crunchwrap Supreme		😊	Free of fructose.
Taco Bell® Mexican Pizza	14½	🍰	Piece (213g); 3089g in total.
Taco Bell® Nachos Supreme		😊	Free of fructose.
Taco, soft corn shell, with beans, cheese	8¼	🍽	Portion (140g); 1155g in total.
Tomato relish		😊	Free of fructose.
Tomato soup mix, dry	6¾	🍽	Portion (34.66g); 234g in total.
Vegetable soup, condensed	B ×¼	😊+	Free of fructose. Per Portion (126g) you eat with it, add B-no × F-limit.
Vichyssoise	B ×¼	😊+	Free of fructose. Per Portion (245g) you eat with it, add B-no × F-limit.
White bean stew with sofrito		😊	Free of fructose.

3.5.2 Meat and fish

Meat and fish	FRUCTOSE	Standard amount
Arby's® Chicken Cordon Bleu Sandwich, crispy	2	Portion (140g); 280g in total.
Beef bacon (kosher)	☺	Free of fructose.
Beef steak, chuck, visible fat eaten	☺	Free of fructose.
Bockwurst	B ×¼ ☺+	Free of fructose. Per Portion (55g) you eat with it, add B-no × F-limit.
Boston Market® 1/4 white rotisserie chicken, with skin	☺	Free of fructose.
Boston Market® roasted turkey breast	☺	Free of fructose.
Bratwurst	B ×¼ ☺+	Free of fructose. Per Portion (55g) you eat with it, add B-no × F-limit.
Bratwurst, beef	B ×1 ☺+	Free of fructose. Per Portion (55g) you eat with it, add B-no × F-limit.
Bratwurst, light (reduced fat)	B ×2¾ ☺+	Free of fructose. Per Portion (55g) you eat with it, add B-no × F-limit.
Bratwurst, made with beer	B ×¼ ☺+	Free of fructose. Per Portion (55g) you eat with it, add B-no × F-limit.
Bratwurst, made with beer, cheese-filled	B ×½ ☺+	Free of fructose. Per Portion (55g) you eat with it, add B-no × F-limit.
Bratwurst, turkey	B ×1½ ☺+	Free of fructose. Per Portion (55g) you eat with it, add B-no × F-limit.
Braunschweiger	☺	Free of fructose.
Caviar	☺	Free of fructose.
Chicken fricassee with gravy, American style	☺	Free of fructose.

Meat and fish	FRUCTOSE	Standard amount
Clams, stuffed with mushroom, onions, and bread	☺	Free of fructose.
Fish croquette	☺	Free of fructose.
Fish sticks, patties, or nuggets, breaded, regular	☺	Free of fructose.
Fish with breading	☺	Free of fructose.
Gorton's® Battered Fish Fillets - Lemon Pepper	☺	Free of fructose.
Gorton's® Popcorn Shrimp, Original	☺	Free of fructose.
Goulash, with beef, noodles or macaroni, tomato base	☺	Nearly free of fructose, avoid at hereditary fructose intolerance.
Herring, pickled	☺	Free of fructose.
Herring, pickled	☺	Free of fructose.
Liver pudding	☺	Free of fructose.
Mrs. Paul's® Calamari Rings	☺	Free of fructose.
Pickled beef	☺	Free of fructose.
Pork cutlet (sirloin cutlet), visible fat eaten	☺	Free of fructose.
Ribs, beef, spare, visible fat eaten	☺	Free of fructose.
Salami, beer or beerwurst, beef	B ×1 ☺+	Free of fructose. Per Portion (55g) you eat with it, add B-no × F-limit.
Salmon, red (sockeye), smoked	☺	Free of fructose.

Meat and fish	FRUCTOSE	Standard amount
Sauerbraten	34¾	Portion (159g); 5525g in total.
Scallops	☺	Free of fructose.
Sea Pak® Seasoned Shrimp, Roasted Garlic	☺	Nearly free of fructose, avoid at hereditary fructose intolerance.
Sea Pak® Shrimp Scampi in Italian Parmesan Sauce	☺	Free of fructose.
Spiced ham loaf (e.g. Spam), canned	☺	Free of fructose.
Tuna, canned, light, oil pack, not drained	☺	Free of fructose.
Venison or deer, stewed	☺	Free of fructose.

3.5.3   Side dishes

Side dishes	FRUCTOSE	Standard amount
Au gratin potato, prepared from fresh	😊	Free of fructose.
Basmati rice, cooked in un-salted water	😊	Free of fructose.
Boston Market® sweet corn	B ×½ 😊+	Free of fructose. Per Portion (85g) you eat with it, add B-no × F-limit.
Bulgur, home cooked	😊	Free of fructose.
Cheese gnocchi	😊	Free of fructose.
Cornbread, from mix	B ×¼ 😊+	Free of fructose. Per Portion (55g) you eat with it, add B-no × F-limit.
Cornbread, homemade	B ×¼ 😊+	Free of fructose. Per Portion (55g) you eat with it, add B-no × F-limit.
Couscous, cooked	😊	Free of fructose.
Falafel	😊	Free of fructose.
Fettuccini noodles, whole wheat, cooked in unsalted water	B ×¼ 😊+	Free of fructose. Per Portion (140g) you eat with it, add B-no × F-limit.
Garbanzo beans (chickpeas), canned, drained	😊	Free of fructose.
Green peas, raw	7¼ 🥄	Tbsp. (15g); 109g in total.
Kidney beans, cooked from dried	😊	Free of fructose.
Lentils, cooked from dried	😊	Free of fructose.
Plain dumplings for stew, biscuit type	😊	Free of fructose.

Side dishes	FRUCTOSE		Standard amount
Polenta	B ×¼	😊 😊+	Free of fructose. Per Portion (240g) you eat with it, add B-no × F-limit.
Potato dumpling (Kartoffelkloesse)	B ×¼	😊 😊+	Free of fructose. Per Portion (140g) you eat with it, add B-no × F-limit.
Potato gnocchi		😊	Free of fructose.
Potato pancakes	B ×½	😊 😊+	Free of fructose. Per Portion (70g) you eat with it, add B-no × F-limit.
Potato, boiled, with skin		😊	Free of fructose.
Potato, boiled, without skin		😊	Free of fructose.
Quinoa, cooked	B ×1¾	😊 😊+	Free of fructose. Per Portion (140g) you eat with it, add B-no × F-limit.
Rice noodles, fried		😊	Free of fructose.
Snow peas (edible pea pods), cooked from fresh	B ×3½	😊 😊+	Free of fructose. Per Portion (85g) you eat with it, add B-no × F-limit.
Spaetzle (spatzen)	B ×¼	😊 😊+	Free of fructose. Per Portion (140g) you eat with it, add B-no × F-limit.

3.6 Fast food chains

3.6.1 Burger King®

Burger King®	FRUCTOSE		Standard amount
Bacon EGG® and Cheese BK Muffin®	B ×1	☺ +	Free of fructose. Per Piece (131g) you eat with it, add B-no × F-limit.
Barbecue sauce	B ×1¼	☺ +	Free of fructose. Per Portion (31g) you eat with it, add B-no × F-limit.
BBQ roasted jalapeno sauce	B ×1	☺ +	Free of fructose. Per Portion (31g) you eat with it, add B-no × F-limit.
BK Big Fish®		☺	Free of fructose.
BK Fresh Apple Slices		☹	Avoid consumption!
BLT Salad® with TenderCrisp chicken (no dressing or croutons)	4¼	🍲	Portion (140g); 595g in total.
Caesar Salad (no dressing or croutons)	1½	🍲	Portion (100g); 150g in total.
Cheeseburger	29½	🍰	Piece (121g); 3570g in total.
French fries		☺	Free of fructose.
Hamburger	32¾	🍰	Piece (109g); 3570g in total.
Ken's® Apple Cider Vinaigrette salad dressing		☺	Free of fructose.
Onion rings	B ×1½	☺ +	Free of fructose. Per Portion (70g) you eat with it, add B-no × F-limit.
Original Chicken Crisp® Sandwich	1½	🍰	Piece (149g); 224g in total.

Burger King®	FRUCTOSE		Standard amount
Pancakes and syrup	B ×6	☺+	Free of fructose. Per Piece (187g) you eat with it, add B-no × F-limit.
Picante taco sauce	2¼		Portion (35g); 79g in total.
Ranch Crispy Chicken Wrap		☺	Free of fructose.
Shake, chocolate	B ×7¼	☺+	Free of fructose. Per Portion (231g) you eat with it, add B-no × F-limit.
Shake, strawberry	B ×5¼	☺+	Free of fructose. Per Portion (229g) you eat with it, add B-no × F-limit.
Shake, vanilla or other	B ×5¾	☺+	Free of fructose. Per Portion (238g) you eat with it, add B-no × F-limit.
Sundaes®, caramel	B ×8½	☺+	Free of fructose. Per Portion (141g) you eat with it, add B-no × F-limit.
Sundaes®, chocolate fudge	B ×6¾	☺+	Free of fructose. Per Portion (141g) you eat with it, add B-no × F-limit.
Sundaes®, mini M & M®	B ×6¾	☺+	Free of fructose. Per Portion (204g) you eat with it, add B-no × F-limit.
Sundaes®, Oreo®	B ×7¼	☺+	Free of fructose. Per Portion (204g) you eat with it, add B-no × F-limit.
Sundaes®, strawberry	B ×2½	☺+	Free of fructose. Per Portion (141g) you eat with it, add B-no × F-limit.
Sweet and sour sauce	¼		Portion (30g); 8g in total.
TenderCrisp® Chicken Sandwich	5		Piece (264g); 1320g in total.
Whopper® with cheese	1¾		Piece (315g); 551g in total.
Zesty onion ring sauce		☺	Free of fructose.

3.6.2 KFC®

KFC®	FRUCTOSE	Standard amount
Caesar salad dressing	😊	Free of fructose.
Chicken breast, spicy crispy	😊	Free of fructose.
Chicken Littles with sauce	3	Piece (101g); 303g in total.
Cole slaw	B ×¼ 😊+	Free of fructose. Per Portion (100g) you eat with it, add B-no × F-limit.
Creamy buffalo sauce	B ×1 😊+	Free of fructose. Per Portion (29.4g) you eat with it, add B-no × F-limit.
Crispy Chicken Caesar Salad	2	Portion (140g); 280g in total.
Crispy Twister without sauce	10¼	Piece (218g); 2235g in total.
Crispy Twister® with sauce	9¼	Piece (240g); 2220g in total.
Extra Crispy Tenders	😊	Free of fructose.
Honey BBQ sauce	B ×1¼ 😊+	Free of fructose. Per Portion (31g) you eat with it, add B-no × F-limit.
Hot wings	😊	Free of fructose.
House side salad	1¾	Portion (100g); 175g in total.
Mashed potatoes with gravy	😊	Free of fructose.
Sweet and sour sauce	¼	Portion (30g); 8g in total.
Sweet corn	😊	Free of fructose.

3.6.3 McDonald's®

McDonald's®	FRUCTOSE	Standard amount
McDonald's® apple Slices	¼	Piece (34g); 9g in total.
McDonald's® Barbecue sauce	B ×1½	Free of fructose. Per Portion (31g) you eat with it, add B-no × F-limit.
McDonald's® Big Mac®	4¼	Piece (215g); 914g in total.
McDonald's® caramel sundae®	B ×6¾	Free of fructose. Per Portion (182g) you eat with it, add B-no × F-limit.
McDonald's® Cheeseburger	3¼	Piece (114g); 371g in total.
McDonald's® Chicken McNuggets®		Free of fructose.
McDonald's® chocolate chip cookies	B ×½	Free of fructose. Per Piece (33g) you eat with it, add B-no × F-limit.
McDonald's® chocolate milk	B ×2	Free of fructose. Per Cup (150 mL) you drink with it, add B-no × F-limit.
McDonald's® Crispy Chicken Snack Wrap with ranch sauce		Free of fructose.
McDonald's® Double Cheese-burger	3½	Piece (165g); 578g in total.
McDonald's® Filet-O-Fish®	1¾	Piece (142g); 249g in total.
McDonald's® French fries		Free of fructose.
McDonald's® Hamburger	3¼	Piece (100g); 325g in total.
McDonald's® hot fudge sun-dae®	B ×7½	Free of fructose. Per Portion (179g) you eat with it, add B-no × F-limit.
McDonald's® hot mustard sauce	B ×1¼	Free of fructose. Per Portion (20g) you eat with it, add B-no × F-limit.

McDonald's®	FRUCTOSE		Standard amount
McDonald's® M & M McFlurry®	B ×3½	☺ +	Free of fructose. Per Portion (228g) you eat with it, add B-no × F-limit.
McDonald's® McCafe shakes, chocolate flavors	B ×5¾	☺ +	Free of fructose. Per Portion (210g) you eat with it, add B-no × F-limit.
McDonald's® McCafe shakes, vanilla or other flavors	B ×¼	☺ +	Free of fructose. Per Portion (206g) you eat with it, add B-no × F-limit.
McDonald's® McChicken®	1½	🍰	Piece (143g); 215g in total.
McDonald's® McDouble®	3½	🍰	Piece (151g); 529g in total.
McDonald's® McRib®	B ×¾	☺ +	Free of fructose. Per Piece (208g) you eat with it, add B-no × F-limit.
McDonald's® Newman's Own® Creamy Caesar salad dressing	39½	🍽	Portion (30g); 1185g in total.
McDonald's® Newman's Own® Low Fat Balsamic Vinaigrette salad dressing		☺	Free of fructose.
McDonald's® orange juice	¾	🥛	Glass (200g); 150 mL in total.
McDonald's® Quarter Pounder	28¾	🍰	Piece (173g); 4974g in total.
McDonald's® Sausage & EGG® McMuffin®	B ×1	☺ +	Free of fructose. Per Piece (164g) you eat with it, add B-no × F-limit.
McDonald's® side salad	2¾	🍽	Portion (100g); 275g in total.
McDonald's® smoothies, all flavors	2½	🥛	Glass (200g); 500 mL in total.
McDonald's® Southwestern chipotle Barbecue sauce	B ×1¾	☺ +	Free of fructose. Per Portion (31g) you eat with it, add B-no × F-limit.
McDonald's® sweet and sour sauce	¼	🍽	Portion (30g); 8g in total.

3.6.4 Subway®

Subway®	FRUCTOSE	Standard amount
9-grain Wheat bread	1	Piece (78g); 78g in total.
American cheese		Free of fructose.
bacon		Free of fructose.
Cheddar cheese		Free of fructose.
Chipotle southwest salad dressing		Free of fructose.
Chocolate chip cookie	B ×1	Free of fructose. Per Piece (45g) you eat with it, add B-no × F-limit.
Chocolate chunk cookie	B ×1	Free of fructose. Per Piece (45g) you eat with it, add B-no × F-limit.
Ham Sandwich with Veggies, no mayo	¾	Piece (219g); 164g in total.
Honey mustard salad dressing	4½	Portion (30g); 135g in total.
Honey Oat bread	2¼	Piece (89g); 200g in total.
Italian BMT® Sandwich with Veggies, no mayo	¾	Piece (226g); 170g in total.
M & M® cookie	B ×½	Free of fructose. Per Piece (45g) you eat with it, add B-no × F-limit.
Mustard		Free of fructose.
Oven Roasted Chicken Sandwich with Veggies, no mayo	1½	Piece (233g); 350g in total.
Parmesan Oregano bread	B ×½	Free of fructose. Per Piece (75g) you eat with it, add B-no × F-limit.

Subway®	FRUCTOSE		Standard amount
Ranch salad dressing		😊	Free of fructose.
Roast Beef Sandwich with Veggies, no mayo	¾		Piece (233g); 175g in total.
Spicy Italian Sandwich with Veggies, no meat	¾		Piece (222g); 167g in total.
Steak & Cheese Sandwich with Veggies, no mayo	¾		Piece (245g); 184g in total.
Sweet Onion Chicken Teri-yaki Sandwich with Veggies, no mayo	12¾		Piece (276g); 3519g in total.
Sweet onion salad dressing	B ×1	😊 +	Free of fructose. Per Portion (30g) you eat with it, add B-no × F-limit.
Tuna Sandwich with Veggies, no mayo	¾		Piece (233g); 175g in total.
Turkey Breast & Ham Sand-wich with Veggies, no mayo	¾		Piece (219g); 164g in total.
Turkey Breast Sandwich with Veggies, no mayo	¾		Piece (219g); 164g in total.
Veggie Delite Salad, no dress-ing	49¾		Portion (100g); 4975g in total.
Veggie Delite Sandwich, no mayo	¾		Piece (162g); 122g in total.
Vinegar		😊	Free of fructose.
White chip macadamia nut cookie		😊	Free of fructose.
Wrap bread		😊	Free of fructose.

3.6.5 Taco Bell®

Taco Bell®	FRUCTOSE		Standard amount
Chalupas Supreme® with beef, beans, cheese	29¾		Portion (140g); 4165g in total.
Taco Bell® Beef Enchirito	2¼		Portion (140g); 315g in total.
Taco Bell® Caramel Apple Empanada	B ×1¼		Free of fructose. Per Portion (125g) you eat with it, add B-no × F-limit.
Taco Bell® Cheesy Fiesta Potatos			Free of fructose.
Taco Bell® cheesy gordita crunch	51		Portion (140g); 7140g in total.
Taco Bell® Cinnamon Twists			Free of fructose.
Taco Bell® Combo Burrito	8¼		Portion (140g); 1155g in total.
Taco Bell® Double Decker Taco Supreme®, beef	25½		Portion (140g); 3570g in total.
Taco Bell® Pintos 'n Cheese	2½		Portion (130g); 325g in total.

3.6.6 Wendy's®

Wendy's®	FRUCTOSE	Standard amount
Strawberry Shake	B ×4¼ 😊+	Free of fructose. Per Glass (200 mL) you drink with it, add B-no × F-limit.
Wendys' chili cheese fries	😊	Free of fructose.
Wendy's® Baconator®	😊	Free of fructose.
Wendy's® Baked Potato, with sour cream and chives	B ×¼ 😊+	Free of fructose. Per Portion (140g) you eat with it, add B-no × F-limit.
Wendy's® Caesar side salad	1¼	Portion (100g); 125g in total.
Wendy's® Chicken Nuggets	😊	Free of fructose.
Wendy's® French fries	😊	Free of fructose.
Wendy's® Frosty Float®	¼	Portion (192g); 48g in total.
Wendy's® Jr. Bacon Cheeseburger	1¾	Portion (140g); 245g in total.
Wendy's® Jr. Cheeseburger Deluxe	3	Portion (140g); 420g in total.
Wendy's® side salad	2¼	Portion (100g); 225g in total.
Wendy's® Spicy Chicken Go Wrap	35½	Portion (140g); 4970g in total.
Wendy's® Spicy Chicken Sandwich	9¾	Portion (140g); 1365g in total.

3.7 Fruits and vegetables

3.7.1 Fruit

Fruit	FRUCTOSE	Standard amount
Apple, fresh, with skin	☹	Avoid consumption!
Applesauce, canned, sweetened	1¼ 🥄	Tbsp. (15g); 19g in total.
Applesauce, canned, unsweetened	¾ 🥄	Tbsp. (15g); 11g in total.
Apricot, dried, cooked, sweetened	B ×1½ ☺+	Free of fructose. Per Piece (20g) you eat with it, add B-no × F-limit.
Apricot, dried, uncooked	B ×8 ☺+	Free of fructose. Per Piece (20g) you eat with it, add B-no × F-limit.
Apricot, fresh	B ×1 ☺+	Free of fructose. Per Piece (35g) you eat with it, add B-no × F-limit.
Banana, chips	3½ 🍽	Portion (40g); 140g in total.
Banana, fresh	B ×¼ ☺+	Free of fructose. Per Piece (118g) you eat with it, add B-no × F-limit.
Blackberries, fresh	3¾ 🍽	Portion (140g); 525g in total.
Blueberries, fresh	3¾ 🍽	Portion (140g); 525g in total.
Boysenberries, fresh	69¼ 🍽	Portion (8g); 554g in total.
Cantaloupe, fresh	1 🍽	Portion (140g); 140g in total.
Carambola (starfruit), fresh	B ×¼ ☺+	Free of fructose. Per Piece (91g) you eat with it, add B-no × F-limit.
Clementine, fresh	7 🍽	Portion (140g); 980g in total.

Fruit	FRUCTOSE		Standard amount
Cranberries, dried (Craisins®)	B ×3¼	☺ +	Free of fructose. Per Portion (40g) you eat with it, add B-no × F-limit.
Cranberries, fresh	B ×2¾	☺ +	Free of fructose. Per Portion (55g) you eat with it, add B-no × F-limit.
Currants, fresh, black	1¼		Portion (140g); 175g in total.
Currants, fresh, red and white	1		Portion (140g); 140g in total.
Dates		☺	Free of fructose.
Elderberries, fresh	¼		Portion (140g); 35g in total.
Figs, dried, cooked, sweetened	B ×¾	☺ +	Free of fructose. Per Piece (50g) you eat with it, add B-no × F-limit.
Figs, fresh	B ×2	☺ +	Free of fructose. Per Piece (50g) you eat with it, add B-no × F-limit.
Gooseberries, fresh	B ×1	☺ +	Free of fructose. Per Portion (140g) you eat with it, add B-no × F-limit.
Grapefruit, fresh, pink or red	2		Portion (140g); 280g in total.
Grapes, fresh	¼		Portion (140g); 35g in total.
Guava (guayaba), fresh, common	1¼		Piece (250g); 313g in total.
Honeydew	¾		Portion (140g); 105g in total.
Jackfruit, fresh		☺	Free of fructose.
Kiwi fruit, gold	1		Piece (86g); 86g in total.
Kiwi fruit, green	3		Piece (69g); 207g in total.

Fruit	FRUCTOSE	Standard amount
Lemon, fresh	😊	Free of fructose.
Lime, fresh	😊	Free of fructose.
Loganberries, fresh	B ×1½ 😊+	Free of fructose. Per Portion (140g) you eat with it, add B-no × F-limit.
Lowbush cranberries (lingonberries)	B ×9¼ 😊+	Free of fructose. Per Portion (140g) you eat with it, add B-no × F-limit.
Lychees (litchis), fresh	1 🥄	Portion (140g); 140g in total.
Lycium (wolf or goji berries)	B ×1 😊+	Free of fructose. Per Portion (140g) you eat with it, add B-no × F-limit.
Mandarin orange, fresh	1¼ 🥄	Portion (140g); 175g in total.
Mango, fresh	1 🥄	Tbsp. (15g); 15g in total.
Mangosteen, fresh	35½ 🥄	Portion (140g); 4970g in total.
Mulberries	½ 🥄	Portion (140g); 70g in total.
Muskmelon	1¼ 🥄	Portion (140g); 175g in total.
Nectarine, fresh	😊	Free of fructose.
Orange, fresh	2¼ 🥄	Portion (140g); 315g in total.
Papaya, fresh	B ×1 😊+	Free of fructose. Per Portion (140g) you eat with it, add B-no × F-limit.
Passion fruit (maracuya), fresh	B ×2½ 😊+	Free of fructose. Per Portion (140g) you eat with it, add B-no × F-limit.
Peach, fresh	B ×1 😊+	Free of fructose. Per Portion (140g) you eat with it, add B-no × F-limit.

Fruit	FRUCTOSE		Standard amount
Pear, fresh	½		Tbsp. (15g); 8g in total.
Persimmon, fresh	2¾		Piece (140g); 385g in total.
Pineapple, dried	½		Portion (40g); 20g in total.
Pineapple, fresh	¾		Portion (140g); 105g in total.
Plantains, green, boiled	¾		Piece (223g); 167g in total.
Plum, fresh	B ×½		Free of fructose. Per Portion (15g) you eat with it, add B-no × F-limit.
Pomegranate, fresh (arils-seed/juice sacs)	B ×½		Free of fructose. Per Piece (15g) you eat with it, add B-no × F-limit.
Quince, fresh	1¼		Tbsp. (15g); 19g in total.
Raisins, uncooked	½		Portion (40g); 20g in total.
Rambutan, canned in syrup	1¼		Portion (140g); 175g in total.
Raspberries, fresh, red	½		Portion (140g); 70g in total.
Rhubarb, fresh			Free of fructose.
Rose hips	B ×½		Free of fructose. Per Portion (140g) you eat with it, add B-no × F-limit.
Santa Claus melon	1¼		Portion (140g); 175g in total.
Sapodilla, fresh	B ×3½		Free of fructose. Per Portion (140g) you eat with it, add B-no × F-limit.
Sour cherries, fresh			Free of fructose.

Fruit	FRUCTOSE		Standard amount
Soursop (guanabana), fresh	1¼		Portion (140g); 175g in total.
Strawberries, fresh	½		Portion (140g); 70g in total.
Sweet cherries, fresh	B ×¼		Free of fructose. Per Portion (15g) you eat with it, add B-no × F-limit.
Watermelon, fresh	1¾		Tbsp. (15g); 26g in total.

3.7.2 Vegetables

Vegetables	FRUCTOSE	Standard amount
Alfalfa sprouts	14½	Portion (85g); 1233g in total.
Artichoke, globe raw	☺	Free of fructose.
Arugula, raw	4¾	Portion (85g); 404g in total.
Asparagus, raw	1½	Portion (85g); 128g in total.
Avocado, green skin, Florida type	B ×1	Free of fructose. Per Portion (30g) you eat with it, add B-no × F-limit.
Bamboo shoots, canned and drained	19½	Portion (85g); 1658g in total.
Beets, raw	☺	Free of fructose.
Black beans, cooked from dried	☺	Free of fructose.
Black olives	☺	Free of fructose.
Bok choy, raw	B ×¼	Free of fructose. Per Portion (85g) you eat with it, add B-no × F-limit.
Boston Market® sweet corn	B ×½	Free of fructose. Per Portion (85g) you eat with it, add B-no × F-limit.
Broccoflower (green cauliflower), cooked from fresh	1	Portion (85g); 85g in total.
Broccoli, raw	3	Portion (85g); 255g in total.
Brown mushrooms (Italian or Crimini mushrooms), raw	B ×¼	Free of fructose. Per Portion (15g) you eat with it, add B-no × F-limit.
Brussels sprouts, cooked from fresh	☺	Free of fructose.
Butternut squash	☺	Free of fructose.

Vegetables	FRUCTOSE		Standard amount
Cabbage, green, cooked	B ×¾	😊+	Free of fructose. Per Portion (85g) you eat with it, add B-no × F-limit.
Cabbage, red, cooked	B ×¼	😊+	Free of fructose. Per Portion (85g) you eat with it, add B-no × F-limit.
Cabbage, savoy, raw		😊	Free of fructose.
Carrots, cooked from fresh		😊	Free of fructose.
Carrots, raw		😊	Free of fructose.
Cauliflower, cooked from frozen		😊	Free of fructose.
Celeriac (celery root), cooked from fresh	6½	🥄	Tbsp. (15g); 98g in total.
Celery, cooked		😊	Free of fructose.
Chard, raw or blanched, marinated in oil	B ×½	😊+	Free of fructose. Per Portion (85g) you eat with it, add B-no × F-limit.
Chayote squash, cooked	6¼	🍽	Portion (130g); 813g in total.
Chestnuts, boiled, steamed		😊	Free of fructose.
Chicory coffee powder, unprepared		😊	Nearly free of fructose, avoid at hereditary fructose intolerance.
Chicory greens, raw	5	🍽	Portion (85g); 425g in total.
Coleslaw, with apples and raisins, mayo dressing	½	🍽	Portion (100g); 50g in total.
Coleslaw, with pineapple, mayo dressing	B ×¼	😊+	Free of fructose. Per Portion (100g) you eat with it, add B-no × F-limit.
Collards, raw		😊	Free of fructose.

Vegetables	FRUCTOSE		Standard amount
Cucumber, raw, with peel	2¾		Portion (85g); 234g in total.
Cucumber, raw, without peel	2½		Portion (85g); 213g in total.
Eggplant, cooked	2¾		Portion (85g); 234g in total.
Endive, curly, raw			Free of fructose.
Enoki mushrooms, raw			Free of fructose.
Fennel bulb, raw	B ×¾		Free of fructose. Per Portion (85g) you eat with it, add B-no × F-limit.
Garbanzo beans (chickpeas), canned, drained			Free of fructose.
Garlic, fresh			Nearly free of fructose, avoid at hereditary fructose intolerance.
Ginger root, raw	89¼		Portion (4g); 357g in total.
Green beans (string beans), cooked from fresh	4½		Portion (85g); 383g in total.
Green bell peppers			Free of fructose.
Green olives			Nearly free of fructose, avoid at hereditary fructose intolerance.
Green tomato, raw	1¾		Portion (85g); 149g in total.
Grits (polenta), regular cooking			Free of fructose.
Hot chili peppers, green, cooked from fresh	4½		Piece (43g); 194g in total.
Hot chili peppers, red, cooked from fresh	2¾		Piece (43g); 118g in total.

Vegetables	FRUCTOSE		Standard amount
Hubbard squash		☺	Free of fructose.
Jerusalem artichoke (sun-choke), raw		☺	Free of fructose.
Kale, raw		☺	Free of fructose.
Kelp, raw		☺	Free of fructose.
Kidney beans, cooked from dried		☺	Free of fructose.
Kohlrabi, cooked	B × ¼	☺	Free of fructose. Per Portion (85g) you eat with it, add B-no × F-limit.
Leeks, leafs	1½		Portion (85g); 128g in total.
Leeks, root	9¼		Tbsp. (15g); 139g in total.
Leeks, whole	1½		Portion (85g); 128g in total.
Lentils, cooked from dried		☺	Free of fructose.
Lettuce, Boston, bibb or butterhead	6¾		Portion (85g); 574g in total.
Lettuce, green leaf	7½		Portion (85g); 638g in total.
Lettuce, iceberg	6		Portion (85g); 510g in total.
Lettuce, red leaf	6¾		Portion (85g); 574g in total.
Lettuce, romaine or cos	1¼		Portion (85g); 106g in total.
Lima beans, cooked from dried	½		Portion (90g); 45g in total.

Vegetables	FRUCTOSE		Standard amount
Lotus root, cooked		☺	Free of fructose.
Maitake mushrooms, raw	B ×½	☺+	Free of fructose. Per Portion (15g) you eat with it, add B-no × F-limit.
Morel mushrooms, raw		☺	Free of fructose.
Mung bean sprouts, cooked from fresh		☺	Free of fructose.
Mung beans, cooked from dried	½	🍲	Portion (90g); 45g in total.
Mushrooms, batter dipped or breaded		☺	Free of fructose.
Okra, raw	2¼	🍲	Portion (85g); 191g in total.
Onion, white, yellow or red, raw		☺	Free of fructose.
Oyster mushrooms, raw	B ×1¾	☺+	Free of fructose. Per Portion (85g) you eat with it, add B-no × F-limit.
Parsnip, cooked	B ×¼	☺+	Free of fructose. Per Portion (85g) you eat with it, add B-no × F-limit.
Pickled beets		☺	Free of fructose.
Portabella mushrooms, cooked from fresh	B ×½	☺+	Free of fructose. Per Portion (15g) you eat with it, add B-no × F-limit.
Purslane, raw	58¾	🍲	Portion (85g); 4994g in total.
Radicchio, raw	2¼	🍲	Portion (85g); 191g in total.
Radish, raw	B ×½	☺+	Free of fructose. Per Portion (85g) you eat with it, add B-no × F-limit.
Rutabaga, raw or blanched, marinated in oil mixture	B ×1	☺+	Free of fructose. Per Portion (85g) you eat with it, add B-no × F-limit.

Vegetables	FRUCTOSE		Standard amount
Sauerkraut		😊	Free of fructose.
Scallop squash	4	🍲	Portion (85g); 340g in total.
Shallot, raw		😊	Free of fructose.
Shiitake mushrooms, cooked	B ×1	😊+	Free of fructose. Per Portion (15g) you eat with it, add B-no × F-limit.
Snow peas (edible pea pods), cooked from fresh	B ×3½	😊+	Free of fructose. Per Portion (85g) you eat with it, add B-no × F-limit.
Sour pickles	B ×¼	😊+	Free of fructose. Per Portion (30g) you eat with it, add B-no × F-limit.
Soybean sprouts, raw		😊	Free of fructose.
Soybeans, cooked from dried	5½	🥄	Tbsp. (15g); 83g in total.
Spaghetti squash	B ×¼	😊+	Free of fructose. Per Portion (85g) you eat with it, add B-no × F-limit.
Spinach, cooked from fresh		😊	Free of fructose.
Split pea sprouts, cooked		😊	Free of fructose.
Straw mushrooms, canned, drained		😊	Free of fructose.
Summer squash, cooked from fresh	2¼	🍲	Portion (85g); 191g in total.
Sun-dried tomatoes, oil pack, drained	½	🥄	Tbsp. (15g); 8g in total.
Sweet potato, boiled		😊	Free of fructose.
Tempeh	3¼	🍲	Portion (85g); 276g in total.

Vegetables	FRUCTOSE	Standard amount
Tomato, cooked from fresh	2¼	Portion (85g); 191g in total.
Turnip, cooked	B ×½	Free of fructose. Per Portion (85g) you eat with it, add B-no × F-limit.
Wax beans (yellow beans), canned, drained		Free of fructose.
Winter melon (waxgourd or chinese preserving melon)		Free of fructose.
Winter type (dark green or orange) squash, cooked	1¾	Portion (130g); 228g in total.
Yams, sweet potato type, boiled		Free of fructose.
Yellow bell pepper, raw	½	Portion (85g); 43g in total.
Yellow tomato, raw	2½	Portion (85g); 213g in total.

3.8 Ice cream

Ice cream	FRUCTOSE		Standard amount
Ben & Jerry's® Ice Cream, Brownie Batter	B ×3	😊+	Free of fructose. Per Portion (110g) you eat with it, add B-no × F-limit.
Ben & Jerry's® Ice Cream, Chocolate Chip Cookie Dough	B ×4¾	😊+	Free of fructose. Per Portion (104g) you eat with it, add B-no × F-limit.
Ben & Jerry's® Ice Cream, Chubby Hubby®	B ×5	😊+	Free of fructose. Per Portion (107g) you eat with it, add B-no × F-limit.
Ben & Jerry's® Ice Cream, Chunky Monkey®	B ×2¾	😊+	Free of fructose. Per Portion (107g) you eat with it, add B-no × F-limit.
Ben & Jerry's® Ice Cream, Half Baked	B ×2¼	😊+	Free of fructose. Per Portion (108g) you eat with it, add B-no × F-limit.
Ben & Jerry's® Ice Cream, Karamel Sutra®	B ×4¾	😊+	Free of fructose. Per Portion (106g) you eat with it, add B-no × F-limit.
Ben & Jerry's® Ice Cream, New York Super Fudge Chunk®	58¾	🍽	Portion (106g); 6228g in total.
Ben & Jerry's® Ice Cream, One Sweet Whirled	B ×4¾	😊+	Free of fructose. Per Portion (106g) you eat with it, add B-no × F-limit.
Ben & Jerry's® Ice Cream, Peanut Butter Cup	B ×5¼	😊+	Free of fructose. Per Portion (115g) you eat with it, add B-no × F-limit.
Ben & Jerry's® Ice Cream, Phish Food®	B ×2¼	😊+	Free of fructose. Per Portion (104g) you eat with it, add B-no × F-limit.
Ben & Jerry's® Ice Cream, Vanilla For A Change	B ×4½	😊+	Free of fructose. Per Portion (103g) you eat with it, add B-no × F-limit.
Breyers® Ice Cream, Natural Vanilla, Lactose Free	B ×4¾	😊+	Free of fructose. Per Portion (65g) you eat with it, add B-no × F-limit.
Dreyer's® Grand Ice Cream, Chocolate	B ×¾	😊+	Free of fructose. Per Portion (65g) you eat with it, add B-no × F-limit.
Dreyer's® No Sugar Added Ice Cream, Triple Chocolate		😊	Free of fructose.

Ice cream	FRUCTOSE		Standard amount
Drumstick® (sundae cone)	B ×2¼	☺ +	Free of fructose. Per Piece (96g) you eat with it, add B-no × F-limit.
Frozen fruit juice Bar	B ×1¼	☺ +	Free of fructose. Per Piece (77g) you eat with it, add B-no × F-limit.
Haagen-Dazs® Desserts Ex-traordinaire Ice Cream, Creme Brulee	B ×4¾	☺ +	Free of fructose. Per Portion (107g) you eat with it, add B-no × F-limit.
Haagen-Dazs® Frozen Yo-gurt, chocolate or coffee fla-vors	B ×¾	☺ +	Free of fructose. Per Portion (106g) you eat with it, add B-no × F-limit.
Haagen-Dazs® Frozen Yo-gurt, vanilla or other flavors	B ×3	☺ +	Free of fructose. Per Portion (106g) you eat with it, add B-no × F-limit.
Haagen-Dazs® Ice Cream, Bailey's Irish Cream	B ×2¾	☺ +	Free of fructose. Per Portion (102g) you eat with it, add B-no × F-limit.
Haagen-Dazs® Ice Cream, Black Walnut	B ×4¾	☺ +	Free of fructose. Per Portion (106g) you eat with it, add B-no × F-limit.
Haagen-Dazs® Ice Cream, Butter Pecan	B ×4¾	☺ +	Free of fructose. Per Portion (106g) you eat with it, add B-no × F-limit.
Haagen-Dazs® Ice Cream, Cherry Vanilla	B ×4½	☺ +	Free of fructose. Per Portion (101g) you eat with it, add B-no × F-limit.
Haagen-Dazs® Ice Cream, Chocolate	B ×2¾	☺ +	Free of fructose. Per Portion (106g) you eat with it, add B-no × F-limit.
Haagen-Dazs® Ice Cream, Coffee	B ×2¾	☺ +	Free of fructose. Per Portion (106g) you eat with it, add B-no × F-limit.
Haagen-Dazs® Ice Cream, Cookies & Cream	B ×4½	☺ +	Free of fructose. Per Portion (102g) you eat with it, add B-no × F-limit.
Haagen-Dazs® Ice Cream, Mango	B ×2¼	☺ +	Free of fructose. Per Portion (106g) you eat with it, add B-no × F-limit.
Haagen-Dazs® Ice Cream, Pistachio	B ×4¾	☺ +	Free of fructose. Per Portion (106g) you eat with it, add B-no × F-limit.
Haagen-Dazs® Ice Cream, Rocky Road	B ×2¾	☺ +	Free of fructose. Per Portion (104g) you eat with it, add B-no × F-limit.

Ice cream	FRUCTOSE		Standard amount
Haagen-Dazs® Ice Cream, Strawberry	B ×4¾	☺ +	Free of fructose. Per Portion (106g) you eat with it, add B-no × F-limit.
Haagen-Dazs® Ice Cream, Vanilla Chocolate Chip	B ×4¾	☺ +	Free of fructose. Per Portion (106g) you eat with it, add B-no × F-limit.
Ice cream sandwich	B ×1½	☺ +	Free of fructose. Per Piece (72g) you eat with it, add B-no × F-limit.
Ice cream, light, no sugar added, with aspartame, vanilla or other flavors (include chocolate chip)		☺	Free of fructose.
Popsicle	B ×1¼	☺ +	Free of fructose. Per Piece (52g) you eat with it, add B-no × F-limit.
Popsicle, sugar free		☺	Free of fructose.
Sorbet, chocolate	B ×3¼	☺ +	Free of fructose. Per Portion (105g) you eat with it, add B-no × F-limit.
Sorbet, coconut	B ×5	☺ +	Free of fructose. Per Portion (106g) you eat with it, add B-no × F-limit.
Sorbet, fruit	B ×5½	☺ +	Free of fructose. Per Portion (106g) you eat with it, add B-no × F-limit.

3.9   Ingredients

Ingredients	FRUCTOSE	Standard amount
Baking powder	😊	Free of fructose.
Barley flour	😊	Free of fructose.
Lemon peel	😊	Free of fructose.
Orange peel	3¼ 🥄	Tbsp. (15g); 49g in total.
Rye flour, in recipes not containing yeast	27¾ 🥄	Portion (30g); 833g in total.
Semolina flour	😊	Free of fructose.
Spelt flour	B ×¼ 😊+	Free of fructose. Per Portion (30g) you eat with it, add B-no × F-limit.
Streusel topping, crumb	😊	Free of fructose.
Wheat bran, unprocessed	😊	Free of fructose.
White all-purpose flour, unenriched	😊	Free of fructose.
White whole wheat flour	33¼ 🥄	Portion (30g); 998g in total.

Glossary

Abbreviation	Meaning
EFSA	European Food Safety Authority.
FDA	Food and Drug Administration.
Fructans	Quickly fermentable carbohydrates that are contained in grain products for example. Included in this group are inulin, kestose and nystose.
Fructose	Oligosaccharide that is primarily contained in fruit.
Galactans	Quickly fermentable carbohydrates that are contained in beans, cabbage, lentils and peas for example (raffinose and stachyose).
Hereditary fructose intolerance	This disease is rare. If you are affected, fructose has a poisonous effect on you. Only a specialist can find out if you are affected and you have to check it before doing a test for fructose intolerance, as it could otherwise be lethal.
Irritable bowel	Definition of this book: an irritable bowel is one that reacts much more intensely to indigestions than it is commonly the case. The presence of trigger cubes in the intestine triggers the symptoms.
Lactose	Oligosaccharide that is primarily contained in dairy products.
Meal	One of three main meals of a given day. The first meal happens at about 7 am the second one at about 1 pm and the third one at about 7 pm. Hence, between each meal there has to be a gap of about six hours in order to avoid overloading your enzyme workers. The tolerable portion sizes refer to this definition of a meal.
NCC	Nutrition Coordination Center of the University of Minnesota.

Abbreviation	Meaning
Sensitivity level	Aside from the standard level, you can use multipliers to determine portion sizes in case you are less sensitive. In the LAXIBA app, we have calculated the tolerable amounts for you. Before increasing your portion sizes to fit another level, you should do a level test to check, if you can tolerate the higher load. There are four levels, see Chapter 3.1.3.
Sorbitol	Sugar alcohol that also limits the tolerated amount of fructose. Besides, see "sugar alcohols".
Standard	Portion sizes in this column are based on the usual sensitivity in case of an intolerance towards to fructose, i.e. as long as you consume less than the stated maximum amount for this level, you are likely to be untroubled by symptoms from it. It only applies in case of intolerance or certain test phases. Note that if you consume the maximum portion size for a food at a meal, you cannot eat any other foods that contain the cube at that meal. To combine two foods that contain a certain cube you have to reduce the stated portion sizes accordingly, e.g. by dividing both by two.
Sugar alcohols	These are contained in some fruit, like apples. Moreover, they are part of many diabetic, dietary and light products as well as chewing gums and mints. They are not contained in stevia. Part of the group of sugar alcohols besides sorbitol are erythritol, inositol, isomalt, lactitol, maltitol, mannitol, pinitol and xylitol.
Trigger(cube)s	Carbohydrates that fermented in the intestine. To this group belong oligosaccharides (fructose, fructans and galactans, lactose) and sugar-alcohols (like sorbitol).

4

ADVANCED PROCEDURES

4.1 Level test

	Level test tasks	✔
1	You filled out the symptom test sheet for the status quo check.	✔
2	You asked your doctor to refer you to a specialist to do a breath test (if available).	✔
3	You performed the three-week introductory diet and found an improvement to your symptoms at the efficiency check (otherwise get *THE IBS NAVIGATOR* and find your trigger). If no breath test was available, you performed the substitute test.	✔
4	Now you convince a partner to help you with your tests. Alternatively, you book a personal trainer at *https://laxiba.com/trainer*. The partner will mix your test liquids and interpret your symptom test sheets. You can count on their confidentiality, credibility and availability.	
5	You finished all of the tests, during which your testing partner adhered to the instructions on page 183, and you acted according to the flowchart on page 194.	
6	Finish: You talked your result over with your testing partner, and adapted your serving sizes to your sensitivity level.	

Each human differs in the amount he or she can stomach of each trigger. Even in healthy humans the tolerated amount of fructose, for example, fluctuates between 5g and 50 g. Moreover, the amount consumed at once for the breath or substitute test is higher than what you would consume in a typical meal. Hence, if your enzyme-workers were able to cope with that amount—you were spared from symptoms after consuming the test does—you can be proud of them, and you can give them a positive interim report: They have mastered all tasks for fructose with flying colors.

If your crew has ached at the dose, at that point all we know is that the extreme test amount has been too much for them. What it does not mean is that the standard portion sizes used in this book are the highest load your enzyme workers can take. Where is your personal threshold up to which you will not have symptoms? To determine it, you use the level test described in the following. With it, you challenge your enzyme worker gradually and check your sensitivity. With each step, you increase the consumption amount of fructose up to the point at which your enzyme workers ask for a pay raise. The flowchart on page 194 on depict the procedure.

For the level test, you ideally have a test partner preparing the test liquids for you and checking the results. If you have one, only let your partner read the instructions on the pages 180 onward. To increase the reliability, you test each level twice. Otherwise, chance could cause something else to trigger your symptom. Should you consider the matter too private and rather not have someone else included, follow the instructions for self-testers you find on those pages.

Start your test week three days before the test day, as symptoms may occur as many as three days after you consume fructose containing foods, and you want to start the check uninfluenced from "old" symptoms. On the days before the test, eat according to your current level. Your current levels the one that you tolerated during the test and retest of the previous test. Initially, it is the standard level, for which you find the serving sizes in the food tables of Chapter 3.

How to run a test week

Day 1–3 before the test day	On the test day	Day 1–3 after
Your cube consumption should undercut your current fructose levels by as narrow a margin as possible, but do not force yourself to eat more of anything than you want. If you do not feel as well on the morning of the test day as you did at the end of the introductory diet, reschedule the test until you do.	Fill out the symptom test sheet on the test day and its three subsequent days.	
	At breakfast, lunch and dinner consume the level dose and apart from that avoid fructose-containing foods.	Eat accoding to the level on day 1-3 before the test. Hence, if you test level 2 go back down to level 1.

Acceleration option: Perform the tests right after one another. Three days after the last test day, begin the next test day and thus save the three days described in the column on the left.

You do not have to fill out the symptom test sheet during the days leading up to the test (page 29). Instead, you can use the efficiency check sheet as your reference, but from the day of the test to the third day after it, document your symptoms (unless you determine an intolerance earlier).

When your testing partner confirms you have an intolerance, the level test is over. You can find the precise procedure in the flowcharts in Section 4.2. A level test of table sugar is unnecessary; you will get the tolerated amount by just multiplying the level amount of tolerated fructose by 10 (see Chapter 3.1.3). For procedural reasons, wait until after you have repeated the test before trying to interpret the results.

How to handle symptoms

After noting discomforts that were so severe that you told your test collaborate you malabsorbed the load, drink water (up to three liters per day are usually healthy) and take a walk to reduce your symptoms.

Information for your level test partner:

My calculated K.O. threshold grade is:

If you want to use the mathematical Option B, presented at the end of this Chapter or are using our downloadable tool, enter your K.O.-grade from the efficiency check above or give your partner the filled out excel sheets. Important: disregard triggers that you can stomach—you can consume products containing them just as you did before. Background: if your estimated symptom grade (lid value) after a level test is lower or equal to the estimate K.O. grade, you have tolerated the test load and thereby the level and otherwise you have not.

 ## Summary

As part of the strategy, you first performed the introductory diet to find out, if the diet did reduce your symptoms after all. If it had an effect, you can go on to determine your individual sensitivity to avoid unnecessary restrictions.

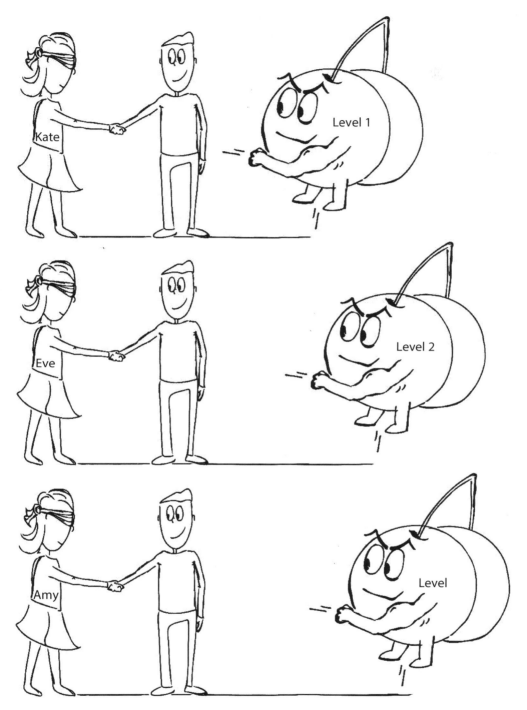

Everyone's sensitivity level is different.

STOP: The following pages are for only your testing partner to read, as they contain information regarding procedural safety—unless you want to do the test alone! Your partner's instructions will depend on your reactions; if you know how your partner is assessing you, you may alter your behavior and distort the results. Continue reading on page 194 to learn about the procedure underlying your partner's tolerance statements. Before and after the three pages for your testing partner are four empty pages. Thus, you can flick back from the end of the book to arrive at page 194 without reading them.

The **instructions** for your testing **partner** follow on page **183**. As the **reader** of the book, you should leave them **unread**, to **produce** a **more accurate** test **result**. Hence, open a new page that is farther **ahead** and then **flick back** to page **194**.

The **instructions** for your testing **partner** follow on page **183**. As the **reader** of the book, you should leave them **unread**, to **produce** a **more accurate** test **result**. Hence, open a new page that is much farther **ahead** and then **flick back** to page **194**.

The **instructions** for your testing **partner** follow on page **183**. As the **reader** of the book, you should leave them **unread**, to **produce** a **more accurate** test **result**. Hence, open a new page that is much farther **ahead** and then **flick back** to page **194**.

The **instructions** for your testing **partner** follow on page **183**. As the **reader** of the book, you should leave them **unread**, to **produce** a **more accurate** test **result**. Hence, open a new page that is much farther **ahead** and then **flick back** to page **194**.

Your friend needs your help! Instructions for testing partners:

You are not the testing partner but the aggrieved party? In case, I caught you! However, of course you also find instructions how to conduct the test yourself. If have a testing partner these lines are not for you, would you please finally move on to page 194!

Now we are in private. Your friend cannot stomach fructose, a common food ingredient, and wants to find out about the personal tolerance limit. Unfortunately, a placebo effect is quite common in this test. Your role in this test is critical for avoiding a false result. You are going to do two rounds for each level, each test taking about a week. On one of the two days, you are going to hand out a placebo mix instead of the real one. Your friend does not know about the placebo. Just say that the double test is required to get valid results, as you also have to keep track of certain behaviors she or he might exhibit. IMPORTANT: Keep quiet about the placebo until **all** tests are done (use the flowcharton page 194) and you have talked the results over. Waiting until the end of that final discussion is important, as your friend may want want to test another level as well. Between two test days are three monitoring days and three regeneration days. Here is what you need: a beaker, a letter scale, and three 0.5 L bottles. Also, instruct your friend to stop taking another bottle if the symptoms after drinking one are already indicating that the load was too much.

> **Note in case you have to do the test without a testing partner:** Prepare the required test bottles on the eve before the test. Make the real and the placebo mix in an equal looking 1-liter-bottle with a non-transparent plastic label (the foil around the bottle on which the brand name shows up). If you use milk, make sure it is still usable for at least two weeks. Now use a pen and write placebo on a colored memo, fold it twice to form a smaller square and put it behind the label of the bottle with the placebo mix. On another note in the same color, you write real mix and put it behind the label of the other bottle. Then you put sticky tape around the tags. Then put both bottles into a non-transparent box that is longer, wider and higher than the bottles. Close it and then turn it around ten times. Thus, you have successfully outwitted yourself: put the bottles in the fridge! On the next morning, you take out one of the bottles, mark it with 1 and drink one third of the mixture in the morning, one third at lunchtime and the rest of the evening (you use one bottle with the daily amount instead of three here, according to the first column of the following tables).

If you find yourself trying to spy at the memo, give yourself a slap on the finger. After the three days following it, where you observed your symptoms, you repeat the test with the other bottle. Again, no fiddling with the label! You have to wait with that until the three observance days of the second bottle are over, too. Now check, how you stomached the placebo versus the real mix.

If your friend has not given you the substances for the test solution, you can order them online or from a pharmacy. You can also ask your pharmacist to weigh the amounts you need. From test to test, increase the level amounts according to the table on the following page. Begin with the level 1 amount. Before repeating the test, note whether you first handed out the real or placebo mix and the result. Ideally, you should ask for the symptom test sheet and write down L for reaL and A for plAcebo as well as the result. Then, keep all of the info sheets for the final discussion of all tests. If your friend has given you the K-grade, you can calculate the tolerance (see row L on page 196). If the L-grade is greater than or equal to K, this indicates an intolerance. There are three possible cases after each double test:

Case 1: Neither the placebo nor the real mix causes the symptoms to worsen, i.e., your friend can stomach the amounts of the ingredient, and you can test the next level. Tell her/him that.

Case 2: Only the real mix causes the symptoms to worsen, i.e., your friend is intolerant for the amount. The test series is over, and you can tell your friend.

Case 3: The placebo mix causes symptoms to worsen. Regardless of whether or not the real mix causes symptoms to worsen, as well, repeat the test with the same amount, starting with the placebo mix, but tell her that you reduced the amount to half of the dose. If your friend still reports an intolerance, abort the test and tell her/him that s/he has an intolerance for the amount, and the old levels remain current.

After the test and retest of the first level, continue according to the level test flowchart on pp. 194. On the eve of one of the two test days, hand out three bottles with the real mix, and on the other one, three bottles with the placebo. At breakfast, lunch and dinner your friend drinks one bottle. Find the mixtures for each level in the following explanation and table:

In the **left column** find the respective **level** and the **total amount** of substances per day, as it is easier to mix the **daily amount in one load** and **then divide** it among the **three bottles**. In the two columns on the right, find the amounts per bottle for the real/placebo substance. Required: fructose and table sugar. Mix the following amounts with 200 mL water and add a little bit of vanilla extract (**v.**). Important: you should not dilute the contents:

Level, real/placebo mix **per day**+600 mL water	Real (R) 3 × 200 mL water bottle with	Placebo (P) 3 × 200 mL water bottle with
Level 1, 3 R/3.5 P, 1 tsp. **v.**	1g fructose 3 drops of **v.**	1.17g sugar 3 drops of **v.**
Level 2, 6 R/7 P, 1 tsp. **v.**	2g fructose 3 drops of **v.**	2.34g sugar 3 drops of **v.**
Level 3, 9 R/10.5 P, 1 tsp. **v.**	3g fructose 3 drops of **v.**	3.51g sugar 3 drops of **v.**

Thank you very much for your support! Even if you have to overcome scruples to knowingly trick your friend… You do not? Well then, enjoy the white lie for good reason!

The **instructions** for your testing **partner** begin on page **183**. As the **reader** of the book, you should leave them **unread**, to **produce** a **more accurate** test **result**. The book resumes on page 194.

The **instructions** for your testing **partner** begin on page **183**. As the **reader** of the book, you should leave them **unread**, to **produce** a **more accurate** test **result**. The book resumes on page 194.

The **instructions** for your testing **partner** begin on page **183**. As the **reader** of the book, you should leave them **unread**, to **produce** a **more accurate** test **result**. The book resumes on page 194.

The **instructions** for your testing **partner** begin on page **183**. As the **reader** of the book, you should leave them **unread**, to **produce** a **more accurate** test **result**.

4.2   Symptom-based test process

The following flow chart shows you the next step, depending on your reaction to the test load. Remember, if you have symptoms after taking the first of three test loads on a test day, abort the test—as this shows that the tested sensitivity level is too high, and there is no point in tantalizing yourself.

You start the test with the first field of the flow chart. The next step always depends on your test result. If you did not stomach a load, the test is over, and you should stick to the level below, which you did tolerate—at the beginning this is the standard amount in the tables in Chapter 3.

All statements assume that you want to perform the level test to the highest level. However, maybe, it is enough to you to know if you tolerate the next level, in the case just stop after the first test. If you do tolerate more than the standard level, note your level next to the multipliers, see Chapter 3.1.3. You will also be able to select your level when using our mobile phone application. Attention: During the combined level tests, you must not pass any level amount that holds for one of your triggers that you do not check at the time as this may otherwise distort the result. If it does happen, you have to repeat the check.

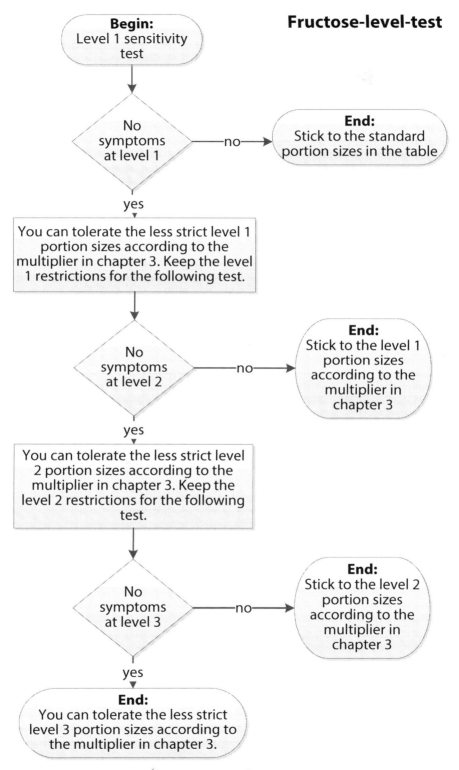

Fructose-level-test

Begin:
Level 1 sensitivity test

No symptoms at level 1

—no→ **End:** Stick to the standard portion sizes in the table

yes

You can tolerate the less strict level 1 portion sizes according to the multiplier in chapter 3. Keep the level 1 restrictions for the following test.

No symptoms at level 2

—no→ **End:** Stick to the level 1 portion sizes according to the multiplier in chapter 3

yes

You can tolerate the less strict level 2 portion sizes according to the multiplier in chapter 3. Keep the level 2 restrictions for the following test.

No symptoms at level 3

—no→ **End:** Stick to the level 2 portion sizes according to the multiplier in chapter 3

yes

End:
You can tolerate the less strict level 3 portion sizes according to the multiplier in chapter 3.

4.3   Test result calculation table

You have two calculation options: option **A** is slightly simpler than option **B**. Real cracks immediately start with **B**. **B** saves time at any further check, and you get a statement on your tolerance. [4]

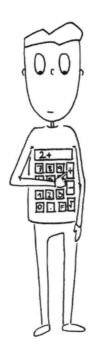

---

[4] From a statistical point of view the survey is slim and the result vague.

4.3.1 The efficiency check calculation table

You use the following table and enter the total intensity of bloating of the respective day into the row **A**. Into the first four cells of that row, you enter the results of the **efficiency check days**, i.e. the last days of your introductory diet. Into the remaining four fields of that row, you enter the values of the **status-quo-days** (the four days before starting your introductory diet, hence, before reducing your trigger consumption).

Calculation option A: Determine $A1$ = total stool grade at the first day of your efficiency check, i.e. your grade in the morning (you calculate your stool grade by multiplying your stool value by the number of defecations you had in the morning) plus the grade at lunchtime plus the grade at the evening. Likewise, you proceed with all other **A**-numbers. Afterward, you determine the **B**-numbers: $B1 = A1$ plus the bloating grade at the first efficiency-check-day plus the pain grade on that day. You calculate $B2$ likewise with the grades for day 2 and so on. Next, you calculate $C2$ and afterward $D2$, which is the average of the status-quo-check-days. To interpret the result, you compare $D2$ with the highest day-grade of the efficiency-check-days, the highest grade of the group $B1$ to $B4$. When checking the success of the introductory diet, it holds that the greater $D2$ lies above the maximum grade of the group the more likely it is that the introductory diet was successful in lowering your symptoms.

Calculation Option B: You calculate $A1$ to $A8$ as well as $B1$ to $B8$ according to the calculation option **A**. Afterward, you estimate $C1$ and $D1$, as well as $C2$ and $D2$ and proceed with the steps described in the table up to K. To interpret the result you compare the $D2$-value with the K-value, i.e. the K. O.[5] threshold grade. At the introductory diet, it holds that: If $D2$ is bigger or equal to the K-grade; this indicates that the diet successfully lowered your symptoms.

If the diet fails, however, get *THE IBS NAVIGATOR* and take the substitute test for fructans and galactans or check alternative triggers as described there.

---

[5] K = if L tops this K.-O.-threshold, the level test amount is too much for your enzyme workers.

	Efficiency check day-				Status-quo-check-day before introductory diet			
	1:	**2:**	**3:**	**4:**	**1:**	**2:**	**3:**	**4:**
A	A1	A3	A3	A4	A5		A6	A7	A8

Enter the total stool grade for each day into the A-cells

B	B1	B2	B3	B4	B5		B6	B7	B8

B5 = stool- + bloating- + pain grade on status-quo-check-day 1

C	C1	$C1 = B1 + B2 + B3 + B4$ Sum of cells B1 to B4 $C2 = B5 + B6 + B7 + B8$ Sum of cells B5 to B8	C2
D	D1	$D1 = C1 \div 4$ Divide your result in cell C1 by 4 $D2 = C2 \div 4$ Divide your result in cell C2 by 4	D2

E	E1	E2	E3	E4	$E1 = B1 - D1, E2 = B2 - D1$ etc. To calculate E1, subtract D1 from B1. Negative results are possible.
F	F1	F2	F3	F4	$F1 = E1 \times E1, F2 = E2 \times E2$ etc. To calculate F1, multiply E1 by itself. As minus times minus is plus, all results are positive.

G	G	$G = F1 + F2 + F3 + F4$ Add your results of the cells F1 to F4
H	H	$H = G \div 4$ Divide G by 4
I	I	I = Take the root of H Take the root of your result in H. On your calculator the root symbol looks like this: $\sqrt{\ }$.
J	J	$J = I \times 2$ Multiply I by 2
K	K	$K = J + D1$ Add the result of cell J to the one in cell D1. The **K**-grade is the **K. O.** threshold grade as the success of the introductory diet depends on it. The diet lowered your symptoms if D2 is bigger than K ($D2 > K$). In addition, you can assess the success of the sensitivity level test with it. You tolerated the tested level if L is not bigger than K ($L \le K$). Please transfer the K-grade to the level test table.

1. Efficiency check calculation with page 31-32 values

	Efficiency-check-day-				Status-quo-check-day before introductory diet			
	1:	**2:**	**3:**	**4:**	**1:**	**2:**	**3:**	**4:**
A	A1	A3	A3	A4	A5	A6	A7	A8
	3	2	3	2	16	14	12	14

Enter the total stool grade for each day into the A-cells

B	B1	B2	B3	B4	B5	B6	B7	B8
	9	8	11	8	30	30	31	28

B5 = stool- + bloating- + pain grade on status-quo-check-day 1

C	C1	C2
	36	119

$C1 = B1 + B2 + B3 + B4$ Sum of cells B1 to B4
$C2 = B5 + B6 + B7 + B8$ Sum of cells B5 to B8

D	D1	D2
	9	29.75

$D1 = C1 \div 4$ Divide your result in cell C1 by 4
$D2 = C2 \div 4$ Divide your result in cell C2 by 4

E	E1	E2	E3	E4
	0	-1	2	-1

$E1 = B1 - D1$, $E2 = B2 - D1$ etc.
To calculate E1, subtract D1 from B1. Negative results are possible.

F	F1	F2	F3	F4
	0	1	4	1

$F1 = E1 \times E1$, $F2 = E2 \times E2$ etc.
To calculate F1, multiply E1 by itself. As minus times minus is plus, all results are positive.

G	G
	6

$G = F1 + F2 + F3 + F4$
Add your results of the cells F1 to F4

H	H
	1.5

$H = G \div 4$
Divide G by 4

I	I
	1.22

$I =$ Take the root of H   Take the root of your result in H. On your calculator the root symbol looks like this: $\sqrt{\ }$.

J	J
	2.45

$J = I \times 2$
Multiply I by 2

K	K
	11.45

$K = J + D1$
Add the result of cell J to the one in cell D1. The *K*-grade is called K. O. threshold grade as the success of the introductory diet ($D2 > K$) and the sensitivity level test ($L \leq K$) depend on it.

Calculation method A

D2 is 29.75 and thus way larger than the highest day grade, 11, (B3) of the group B1 to B4, which indicates the success of the introductory diet.

Calculation method B

D2 = 29.75 is bigger than K = 11.45, and that shows the success of the diet. Had D2 been smaller or equal to K, , get *THE IBS NAVIGATOR* and check other triggers.

4.3.2 The level test calculation table

Use the following table and enter the grades of the level test days. You only need to estimate the grades from the level test sheet (enter them into B5 to B8. If you used math option B, just enter the K value, and you are ready to determine your result. If you use math option A, you have to calculate D1. Having done the introductory diet is, of course, necessary.

Calculation option A: *A1* = stool grade at the first efficiency-check-day, i.e. grade in the morning (multiply the stool value in the morning by the number of defecations you had in the morning) plus stool grade at lunchtime plus stool grade at the evening. Enter your total stool grade into the cell with the *A1* in italic. Likewise, you proceed with all other **A**-Numbers. Afterward, estimate the **B-grades**: *B1* = *A1* plus total bloating grade, plus total pain grade on the test day. You calculate *B2* with the grades for the first day after the test day and so on. Next, you determine *C1* and afterward *D1*, i.e. the average of the efficiency-check days. To interpret the result, compare *D1* with the highest day grade of the level test days, *B5* to *B8*. When checking the success of the diet, it holds that the much greater the largest day grade is compared to *D1*, the rather you did not tolerate the load of the tested sensitivity level. If that is the case, stick to the portion sizes of a lower sensitivity level.

Calculation option B: If you calculated *K* at the efficiency check—you should have as doing a level test before checking the efficiency of the diet makes no sense—just copy it to this table. Aside from it, all you need is to estimate *B1* to *B8* according to calculation option **A** and determine *L*. For the assessment, you compare the *L*-, i.e. the level grade with the *K*-grade, the K.-O.-threshold grade. It holds: if *L* is bigger than *K*, this means that the amount consumed during the test has triggered symptoms. Therefore, you should stick to the portion sizes of the sensitivity level below at which your symptoms improved. If *L* is lower than *K*, you tolerated the level amount and can have the less restricted diet according to that level. What is more, you can check an even higher sensitivity level if you want.

	Efficiency-check-day-				Level-test	day after test day-		
	1:	**2:**	**3:**	**4:**	**Test day**	**1:**	**2:**	**3:**
A	A1	A3	A3	A4	A5	A6	A7	A8

Enter the total stool grade for each day into the A-cells

B	B1	B2	B3	B4	B5	B6	B7	B8

B5 = stool- + bloating- + pain grade on status-quo-check-day 1

C	C1	$C1 = B1 + B2 + B3 + B4$ Sum of the cells B1 to B4
D	D1	$D1 = C1 \div 4$ Divide your results in cell C1 by 4
K	K	*Please copy the K grade you estimated at the end of the introductory diet to this field. If you have not yet calculated it, do it now as described in the efficiency-check-calculation-table.*
L	L	L = is the biggest grade of the group: B5, B6, B7, B8. This group contains the results of the level test day (B5) and the three days following it (B6 to B8). With the L-grade, you evaluate the current Level test. Assessment: $L > K$, if L is bigger than K, it means that the tested load for that level caused you symptoms and that you, therefore, should adjust your diet to a lower sensitivity level. $L \leq K$, if L is lower or equal to K, it means that you tolerated the load of that level per meal.

1. Level test calculation with the page 31-32 values

	Efficiency-check-day-				Level-test	day after test day-		
	1:	**2:**	**3:**	**4:**	**Test day**	**1:**	**2:**	**3:**
A	A1	A3	A3	A4	A5	A6	A7	A8
	3	2	3	2	16	14	12	14

Enter the total stool grade for each day into the A-cells

B	B1	B2	B3	B4	B5	B6	B7	B8
	9	8	11	8	30	30	31	28

B5 = stool- + bloating- + pain grade on status-quo-check-day 1

C	C1	C1 = B1 + B2 + B3 + B4 Sum of the cells B1 to B4
	36	
D	D1	D1 = C1 ÷ 4 Divide your results in cell C1 by 4
	9	
K	K	Please copy the K grade you estimated at the end of the introductory diet to this field. If you have not yet calculated it, do it now as described in the *efficiency-check-calculation-table*.
	11.45	
L	L	L = is the biggest grade of the group: B5, B6, B7, B8. This group contains the results of the level test day (B5) and the three days following it (B6 to B8). With the L-grade, you evaluate the current Level test. Assessment:
		L > K, if L is bigger than K, it means that the tested load for that level caused you symptoms and that you, therefore, should adjust your diet to a lower sensitivity level.
	31	L ≤ K, if L is lower or equal to K, it means that you tolerated the load of that level per meal.

Calculation method A

The highest total grade of a day of the group B5 to B8, B7 = 31 is way above D1 = 9, which indicates that you did not tolerate the level amount. If the highest grade of the group B5 to B8 had been smaller or equal to 9, you would have tolerated the sensitivity level amount and could have taken a less restricted diet according to the amounts of that level. Moreover, you could have tested the next level for people that are even less sensitive.

Calculation method B

As L = 31 is bigger than K = 11.45, you have not tolerated the level load of that trigger. Had L been smaller or equal to 11.45, you would have endured the level amount and could have followed the less strict diet for that level. Moreover, you could have tested the next higher tolerance level.

Sources

Ali, M., Rellos, P., & Cox, T. M. (1998). Heriditary fruktose intolerance. *Journal of Medical Genetics*, 35(5), 353-365.

American Cancer Society (2015). *Colorectal cancer and early detection.* Retrieved from: www.cancer.org/acs/groups/cis/documents/webcontent/003170-pdf.pdf.

Ananthakrishnan, A. N., Higuchi, L. M., Huang, E. S., Khalili, H., Richter, J. M., Fuchs, C. S., & Chan, A. T. (2012). Aspirin, nonsteroidal anti-inflammatory drug use, and risk for Crohn disease and ulcerative colitis: a cohort study. *Annals of Internal Medicine*, 156(5), 350-359.

Barrett, J. S., Gearry, R. B., Muir, J. G., Irving, P. M., Rose, R., Rosella, O., ... & Gibson, P. R. (2010). Dietary poorly absorbed, short-chain carbohydrates increase delivery of water and fermentable substrates to the proximal colon. *Alimentary Pharmacology & Therapeutics*, 31(8), 874-882.

Balasubramanya, N. N., Sarwar, & Narayanan, K. M. (1993). Effect of stage of lactation on oligosaccharides level in milk. *Indian Journal of Dairy & Biosciences*, 4, 58-60.

Belitz, H.-D., Grosch, W., & Schieberle, P. (2008). *Lehrbuch der Lebensmittelchemie* (6th ed.). Berlin Heidelberg: Springer.

Berekoven, L., Eckert, W., Ellenrieder, P. (2009). Marktforschung: *Methodische Grundlagen und praktische Anwendung* (12th ed.). Wiesbaden: Gabler.

Bernstein, C. N., Fried, M., Krabshuis, J. H., Cohen, H., Eliakim, R., Fedail, S., ... & Watermeyer, G. (2010). World Gastroenterology Organization Practice Guidelines for the diagnosis and management of IBD in 2010. *Inflammatory Bowel Diseases*, 16(1), 112-124.

Biesiekierski, J. R., Rosella, O., Rose, R., Liels, K., Barrett, J. S., Shepherd, S. J., ... & Muir, J. G. (2011). Quantification of fructans, galacto-oligosacharides and other short-chain carbohydrates in processed grains and cereals. *Journal of Human Nutrition and Dietetics*, 24(2), 154-176.

Binnendijk, K. H., & Rijkers, G. T. (2013). What is a health benefit? An evaluation of EFSA opinions on health benefits with reference to probiotics. *Beneficial Microbes*, 4(3), 223-230.

Blumenthal, M. (1998). *The Complete German Commission E Monographs; Therapeutic Guide to Herbal Medicine*. Boston, MA: Integrative Medicine Communications.

Boehm, G., & Stahl, B. (2007). Oligosaccharides from milk. *The Journal of Nutrition,* 137(3), 847S-849S.

Bowden, P. (2011). *Telling It Like It Is.* Paul Bowden.

Briançon, S., Boini, S., Bertrais, S., Guillemin, F., Galan, P., & Hercberg, S. (2011). Long-term antioxidant supplementation has no effect on health-related quality of life: The randomized, double-blind, placebo-controlled, primary prevention SU.VI.MAX trial. *International Journal of Epidemiology,* 40(6), 1605-1616.

Campbell, J. M., Fahey, G. C., & Wolf, B. W. (1997). Selected indigestible oligosaccharides affect large bowel mass, cecal and fecal short-chain fatty acids, pH and microflora in rats. *The Journal of Nutrition,* 127(1), 130-136.

Chi, W. J., Chang, Y. K., & Hong, S. K. (2012). Agar degradation by microorganisms and agar-degrading enzymes. *Applied Microbiology and Biotechnology,* 94(4), 917-930.

Choi, Y. K; Johlin Jr., F. C.; Summers, R.W., Jackson, M., & Rao, S. S. C. (2003). Fruktose intolerance: an under-recognized problem. *The American Journal of Gastroenterology,* 98(6) 2003, S. 1348-1353.

CIAA (n. d.). *CIAA agreed reference values for GDAs* [Table]. Retrieved from http://gda.fooddrinkeurope.eu/asp2/gdas_portions_rationale.asp?doc_id=127.

Connor, W. E. (2000). Importance of n− 3 fatty acids in health and disease. *The American Journal of Clinical nutrition,* 71(1), 171S-175S.

Coraggio, L. (1990). *Deleterious Effects of Intermittent Interruptions on the Task Performance of Knowledge Workers: A Laboratory Investigation* (Doctoral Dissertation). Retrieved from http://arizona.openrepository.com.

Corazza, G. R., Strocchi, A., Rossi, R., Sirola, D., & Fasbarrini, G. (1988). Sorbitol malabsorption in normal volunteers and in patients with celiac disease. *Gut,* 29(1), 44-48.

Cummings, J. H. (1981). Short chain fatty acids in the human colon. *Gut,* 22(9), 763-779.

Cummings, J. H., & Macfarlane, G. T. (1997). Role of intestinal bacteria in nutrient metabolism. *Journal of Parental and Enteral Nutrition,* 21(6), 357-365.

DGE (2013). Vollwertig essen und trinken nach den 10 Regeln der DGE. 9th Edition, Bonn.

Donker, G. A., Foets, M., & Spreeuwenberg, P. (1999). Patients with irritable bowel syndrome: health status and use of healthcare services. *British Journal of General Practice,* 49(447), 787-792.

Drossman, D. A., Li, Z., Andruzzi, E., Temple, R. D., Talley, N. J., Thompson, W. G. …Corazziari, E. et al. (1993). US householder survey of functional gastrointestinal disorders: prevalence, sociodemography, and health impact. *Digestive Diseases and Sciences*, 38(9), 1569-1580.

Dukas, L., Willett, W. C., & Giovannucci, E. L. (2003). Association between physical activity, fiber intake, and other lifestyle variables and constipation in a study of women. *The American Journal of Gastroenterology*, 98(8), 1790-1796.

EFSA (2007). Opinion of the scientific panel on dietetic products, nutrition and allergies on a request from the commission related to a notification from epa on lactitol pursuant to article 6, paragraph 11 of directive 2000/13/ec- for permanent exemption from labeling. *The EFSA Journal*, 5(10), 565-570.

EFSA (2012a). Scientific opinion on dietary reference values for protein. *The EFSA Journal*, 10(2), 2557-2622.

EFSA (2012b). Scientific opinion on the substantiation of health claims related to lactobacillus casei dg cncm i-1572 and decreasing potentially pathogenic gastro-intestinal microorganisms (id 2949, 3061, further assessment) pursuant to article 13(1) of regulation (ec) no 1924/2006. *The EFSA Journal*, 10(6), 2723-2637.

EFSA (2012c). Scientific opinion on the tolerable upper intake level of eicosapentaenoic acid (epa), docosahexaenoic acid (dha) and docosapentaenoic acid (dpa). *The EFSA Journal*, 10(7), 2815-2862.

EFSA (2013). scientific opinion on the substantiation of a health claim related to bimuno® gos and reducing gastro-intestinal discomfort pursuant to article 13(5) of regulation (ec) no 1924/2006. *The EFSA Journal*, 11(6), 3259-3268.

Eisenführ, F., Weber, M., & Langer, T. (2010): *Rational Decision Making*, Heidelberg, Berlin: Springer.

Erdman, K., Tunnicliffe, J., Lun, V. M., & Reimer, R. A. (2013). Eating patterns and composition of meals and snacks in elite canadian athletes. *International Journal Of Sport Nutrition & Exercise Metabolism*, 23(3), 210-219.

Evans, J. M., McMahon, A. D., Murray, F. E., McDevitt, D. G., & MacDonald, T. M. (1997). Non-steroidal anti-inflammatory drugs are associated with emergency admission to hospital for colitis due to inflammatory bowel disease. *Gut*, 40(5), 619-622.

Falony, G., Verschaeren, A. De Bruycker, F., De Preter, V., Verbecke, F. L., & De Vuyst L. (2009b). In vitro kinetics of prebiotic inulin-type fructan fermentation by butyrate-producing colon bacteria: implementation of online gas chromatography for quantitative analysis of carbon dioxide and hydrogen gas production. *Applied Environmental Microbiology*, 75(18), 5884-5892.

FAO (2008). Fats and fatty acids in human nutrition. *FAO Food and Nutrition Paper*, 91, 9-20.

Farquhar, P. H., & Keller, L. R. (1989). Preference intensity measurement. *Annals of Operations Research*, 19(1), 205-217.

Farshchi, H. R., Taylor, M. A., & Macdonald, I. A. (2004). Regular meal frequency creates more appropriate insulin sensitivity and lipid profiles compared with irregular meal frequency in healthy lean women. *European Journal of Clinical Nutrition*, 58(7), 1071-1077.

Fasano, A., & Catassi, C. (2001). Current approaches to diagnosis and treatment of celiac disease: an evolving spectrum. *Gastroenterology*, 120(3), 636-651.

Fass, R., Fullerton, S., Naliboff, B., Hirsh, T., & Mayer, E. A. (1998). Sexual dysfunction in patients with irritable bowel syndrom and non-ulcer dyspepsia. *Digestion*, 59(1), 79-85.

Fernández-Bañares, F., Esteve-Pardo, M., de Leon, R., Humbert, P., Cabré, E., Llovet, J. M., & Gassull, M. A. (1993). Sugar malabsorption in functional bowel disease: clinical implications. *American Journal of Gastroenterology*, 88(12), 2044-2050.

Fox, K. (2013). N. t.. In Wells, V., Wyness, L., & Coe, S. (Eds.). The British Nutrition Foundation's 45th anniversary conference: behaviour change in relation to healthier lifestyles. *Nutrition Bulletin*, 38(1), 100-107.

Gaby, A. R. (2005). Adverse effects of dietary fruktose. *Alternative medicine review*, 10(4).

Gay-Crosier, F., Schreiber, G., & Hauser, C. (2000). Anaphylaxis from inulin in vegetables and processed food. *The New England Journal of Medicine*, 342(18), 1372.

German, J., Freeman, S., Lebrilla, C., & Mills, D. (2008). Human milk oligosaccharides: evolution, structures and bioselectivity as substrates for intestinal bacteria, *Nestlé Nutrition Workshop, Pediatric Program*, 62, 205-222.

Gibson, P. R., Newnham, E., Barrett, J. S., Shepherd, S. J., & Muir, J. G. (2007). Review article: Fruktose malabsorption and the bigger picture. *Alimentary Pharmacology & Therapeutics*, 25(4), 349-363.

Gibson, P. R., & Shepherd, S. J. (2010). Evidence-based dietary management of functional gastrointestinal symptoms: the fodmap approach. *Journal of Gastroenterology and Hepatology*, 25(2), 252-258.

Gilbert, P. (2013). N. t.. In Wells, V., Wyness, L., & Coe, S. (Eds.). The British Nutrition Foundation's 45th anniversary conference: behaviour change in relation to healthier lifestyles. *Nutrition Bulletin*, 38(1), 100-107.

Goldstein, R., Braverman, D., & Stankiewicz, H. (2000). Carbohydrate malabsorption and the effect of dietary restriction on symptoms of irritable bowel syndrome and functional bowel complaints. *Israel Medical Association Journal*, 2(8), 583-587.

Gralnek, I. M., Hays, R. D., Kilbourne, A., Naliboff, B., & Mayer, E. A. (2000). The impact of irritable bowel syndrome on health-related quality of life. *Gastroenterology*, 119(3), 654-660.

Hahn, B. A., Kirchdoerfer, L. J., Fullerton, S., & Mayer, S. (1997). Patient perceived severity of irritable bowel syndrome in relation to symptoms, health resource utilization and quality of life. *Alimentary Pharmacology and Therapeutics*, 11(3), 553-559.

Hallert, C., Grant, C., Grehn, S., Grännö, C., Hultén, S., Midhagen, G., ... & Valdimarsson, T. (2002). Evidence of poor vitamin status in coeliac patients on a gluten-free diet for 10 years. *Alimentary Pharmacology & Therapeutics*, 16(7), 1333-1339.

Hanauer, S. B. (2006). Inflammatory bowel disease: epidemiology, pathogenesis, and therapeutic opportunities. *Inflammatory Bowel Diseases*, 12(5), S3-S9.

Hawthorne, B., Lambert, S., Scott, D., & Scott, B. (1991). Food intolerance and the irritable bowel syndrome. *Journal of Human Nutrition and Dietetics*, 4(1), 19–23.

Hawking, S. (n. d.). *Publications*. Retrieved from http://hawking.org.uk/publications.html.

Hillson, M. (2013). N. t.. In Wells, V., Wyness, L., & Coe, S. (Eds.). The British Nutrition Foundation's 45th anniversary conference: behaviour change in relation to healthier lifestyles. *Nutrition Bulletin*, 38(1), 100-107.

Hoekstra, J. H., van Kempen, A. A. M. W., & Kneepkens, C. M. F. (1993). Apple juice malabsorption: fruktose or sorbitol?. *Journal of Pediatric Gastroenterology and Nutrition*, 16(1), 39-42.

Huether, G. (Lecturer) (2014*). Interview mit Prof. Dr. Gerald Hüther zu Angst & Berufung*. Retrieved from http://www.coach-your-self.tv/Startseite/TV/InterviewmitProfDrH%c3%BctherzuAngstBerufung/tabid/1341/Default.aspx

Hyams, J. S. (1983). Sorbitol intolerance: an unappreciated cause of functional gastrointestinal complaints. *Gastroenterology*, 84(1)1, 30-33.

Hyams, J. S., Etienne, N. L., Leichtner, A. M., & Theuer, R. C. (1988). Carbohydrate malabsorption following fruit juice ingestion in young children. *Pediatrics*, 82(1), 64-68.

Itzkowitz, S. H. & Daniel, H. (2005). Concensus Coference: colorectal cancer screening and surveillance in inflammatory bowel disease. *Inflammatory Bowel Disease*, 11(3).

Jameson, S. (2000). Coeliac disease, insulin-like growth factor, bone mineral density, and zinc. *Scandinavian Journal of Gastroenterology*, 35(8), 894-896.

Jemal, A., Siegel, R., Ward, E., Murray, T., Xu, J. Smigal, C., & Thun, M. J. (2006). Cancer statistics, 2006. *CA: A Cancer Journal for Clinicians*, 56(2), 106-130.

Jensen, R. G., Blanc, B., & Patton, S. (1995). Particulate constituents in human and bovine milks. In Jensen, R. G. (Ed.), *Handbook of Milk Composition* (pp. 51-62). San Diego: Academic Press.

Kennedy, E. (2004). Dietary diversity, diet quality, and body weight regulation. *Nutrition Reviews*, 62(s2), S78-S81.

Kneepkens, C. M. F., Vonk, R. J., & Fernandes, J. (1984). Incomplete intestinal absorption of fruktose. *Archives of Disease in Childhood*, 59(8), 735-738.

Kneepkens, C. M. F., Jakobs, C., & Douwes, A. C. (1989): Apple juice, fruktose, and chronic nonspecific diarrhoea. *Pediatrics*, 148(6), 571-573.

Knudsen, B. K., & Hessov, I. (1995). Recovery of inulin from Jerusalem artichoke (Helianthus tuberosus L.) in the small intestine of man. *British Journal of Nutrition*, 74(01), 101-113.

Komericki, P., Akkilic-Materna, M., Strimitzer, T., Weyermair, K., Hammer, H. F., & Aberer, W. (2012). Oral xylose isomerase decreases breath hydrogen excretion and improves gastrointestinal symptoms in fruktose malabsorption – a double-blind, placebo-controlled study. *Alimentary Pharmacology & Therapeutics*, 36(10), 980-987.

Kornbluth, A., & Sachar, D. B. (2004). Ulcerative colitis practice guidelines in adults (update): American College of Gastroenterology, Practice Parameters Committee. *The American Journal of Gastroenterology*, 99(7), 1371-1385.

Kuhn, R., & Gauhe, A. (1965). Bestimmung der bindungsstelle von sialinsäureresten in oligosacchariden mit hilfe von perjodat. *Chemische Berichte*, 98(2), 395-314.

Kupper, C. (2005). Dietary guidelines and implementation for celiac disease. *Gastroenterology*, 128(4), 121-127.

Kushi, L. H., Doyle, C., McCullough, M., Rock, C. L., Demark-Wahnefried, W. Bandera, E. V., ... & Gansler, T. (2012). American cancer society guidelines on nutrition and physical activity for cancer prevention. *CA: A Cancer Journal for Clinicians*, 62(1), 30-67.

Ladas, S. D., Grammenos, I., Tassios, P. S., & Raptis, S. A. (2000). Coincidental malabsorption of laktose, fruktose, and sorbitol ingested at low doses is not Common in normal adults. *Digestive Diseases and Sciences*, 45(12), 2357-2362.

Langkilde, A. M., Andersson, H., Schweizer, T. F., & Würsch, P. (1994). Digestion and absorption of sorbitol, maltitol and isomalt from the small bowel. A study in ileostomy subjects. *European Journal of Clinical Nutrition*, 48(11), 768-775.

Latulippe, M. E., & Skoog, S. M. (2011). Fruktose malabsorption and intolerance: effects of fruktose with and without simultaneous glucose ingestion. *critical Reviews in Food Science and Nutrition*, 51(7), 583-592.

Le, A. S., & Mulderrig, K. B. (2001). *Sorbitol and Mannitol*. Nabors, O'B. (Ed.). New York, NY: Marcel Dekker.

Ledochowski, M., Sperner-Unterweger, B., Widner, B., & Fuchs, D. (1998a). Fruktose malabsorption is associated with early signs of mentral depression. *European Journal of Medical Research*, 3(6), 295-298.

Ledochowski, M., Sperner-Unterweger, B., & Fuchs, D. (1998b). Laktose malabsorption is associated with early signs of mental depression in females – a preliminary report. *Digestive Diseases and Sciences*, 43(11), 2513-2517.

Ledochowski, M., Überall, F., Propst, T., & Fuchs, D. (1999). Fruktose malabsorption is associated with lower plasma folic acid concentrations in middle-aged subjects. *Clinical Chemistry*, 45(11), 2013-2014.

Ledochowski, M., Widner, B., Bair, H., Probst, T., & Fuchs, D. (2000a). Fruktose-and sorbitol-reduced diet improves mood and gastrointestinal disturbances in fruktose malabsorbers. *Scandinavian Journal of Gastroenterology*, 35(10), 1048-1052.

Ledochowski, M., Widner, B., Sperner-Unterweger, B., Probst, T., Vogel, W., & Fuchs, D. (2000b). Carbohydrate malabsobtion syndromes and early signs of mental depression in females. *Digestive Diseases and Sciences*, 45(12), 1255-1259. [Anm. d. Verf.: Die Studie ist für Männer nicht aussagekräftig, da die Stichprobengröße zu klein ist.]

Leinoel (n. d.). *Leinöl(Leinsamen)*. Retrieved from http://www.vitalstoff-journal.de/vitalstoff-lexikon/l/leinoel-leinsamen.

Lewis, S. J., & Heaton, K. W. (1997). Stool form scale as a useful guide to intestinal transit time. *Scandinavian Journal of Gastroenterology*, 32(9), 920-924.

Lifschitz, C. H. (2000). Carbohydrate absorption from fruit juices in infants. *Pediatrics*, 105(1), e4.

Lombardi, D. A., Jin, K., Courtney, T. K., Arlinghaus, A., Folkard, S., Liang, Y., & Perry, M. J. (2014). The effects of rest breaks, work shift start time, and sleep on the onset of severe injury among workers in the People's Republic of China. *Scandinavian Journal of Work, Environment & Health*, 40(2), 146-155.

Lomer, M. C. E., Parkes, G. C., & Sanderson, J. D. (2008). Review article: Lactose intolerance in clinical practice – myths and realities. *Alimentary Pharmacology & Therapeutics*, 27(2), 93-103.

Longstreth, G. F., Thompson, W. G., chey, W. D., Houghton, L. A., Mearin, F., & Spiller, R. C. (2006). Functional bowel disorders. *Gastroenterology*, 130(5), 1480-1491.

Maintz, L., & Novak, N. (2007). Histamine and histamine intolerance. *The American Journal of Clinical Nutrition*, 85(5), 1185-1196.

Makras, L., Van Acker, G., & De Vuyst, L. (2005). Lactobacillus paracasei subsp. paracasei 8700: 2 degrades inulin-type fructans exhibiting different degrees of polymerization. *Applied and Environmental Microbiology*, 71(11), 6531-6537.

Mccoubrey, H., Parkes, G. C., Sanderson, J. D., & Lomer, M. C. E. (2008). Nutritional intakes in irritable bowel syndrome. *Journal of Human Nutrition and Dietetics*, 21(4), 396-397.

McKenzie, Y. A., Alder, A., Anderson, W. Goddard, L, Gulia, P., Jankovich, E. ...Lomer, M. C. E. (2012). British dietic association evidence-based guidelines for the dietary management of irritable bowel syndrome in adults. *Journal of Human Nutrition and Dietics*, 25(3), 260-274.

Meyrand, M., Dallas, D. C., caillat, H., Bouvier, F., Martin, P., & Barile, D. (2013). Comparison of milk oligosaccharides between goats with and without the genetic ability to synthesize αs1-casein. *Small Ruminant Research*, 113(2), 411-420.

Michel, G., Nyval-Collen, P., Barbeyron, T., czjzek, M., & Helbert, W. (2006). Bioconversion of red seaweed galactans: a focus on bacterial agarases and Carrageenases. *Applied Microbiology and Biotechnology*, 71(1), 23-33.

Michie, S. (2013). N. t.. In Wells, V., Wyness, L., & Coe, S. (Eds.). The British Nutrition Foundation's 45th anniversary conference: Behaviour change in relation to healthier lifestyles. *Nutrition Bulletin*, 38(1), 100-107.

Mishkin, D., Sablauskas, L., Yalovsky, M., & Mishkin, S. (1997). Fruktose and sorbitol malabsorption in ambulatory patients with functional dyspepsia: comparison with laktose maldigestion/malabsorption. *Digestive Diseases and Sciences*, 42(12), 2591-2598.

Molodecky N. A., Soon, I. S., Rabi, D. M., et al. (2012). Increasing incidence and precalence of the inflammatory bowel diseases with time, based on systematic review. *Gastroenterology*, 142(1), 46-54.

Monash University (2014). *The Monash University Low Foodmap Diet* [Software]. Available from http://www.med.monash.edu/cecs/gastro/fodmap/education.html

Montalto, M., Curigliano, V., Santoro, L., Vastola, M., Cammarota, G., Manna, R., ... & Gasbarrini, G. (2006). Management and treatment of laktose malabsorption. *World Journal of Gastroenterology*, 12(2), 187.

Molis, C., Flourié, B., Ouarne, F., Gailing, M. F., Lartigue, S., Guibert, A., Bornet, F., & Galmiche, F. P. (1996). Digestion, excretion, and energy value of fructooligosaccharides in healthy humans. *The American Society for Clinical Nutrition*, 64(3), 324-328.

Mosby's Medical Dictionary (8th ed.). St. Louis, MO: Mosby.

Moshfegh, A. J., James, E. F., Goldman, J. P., & Ahuja, J. L. C. (1999). Presence of inulin and oligofruktose in the diets of Americans. *The Journal of Nutrition*, 129(7), 1407S-1411S.

Mount Sinai (n. d.). *Fiber Chart*. Retrieved from https://www.wehealny.org/healthinfo/dietaryfiber/fibercontentchart.html.

Mozaffarian, D., & Wu, J. H. (2011). Omega-3 fatty acids and cardiovascular disease effects on risk factors, molecular pathways, and clinical events. *Journal of the American College of Cardiology*, 58(20), 2047-2067.

Muir, J. G., Shepherd, S. J., Rosella, O., Rose, R., Barrett, J. S., & Gibson, P. R. (2007). Fructan and free fruktose content of common Australian vegetables and fruit. *Journal of Agricultural and Food Chemistry*, 55(16), 6619-6627.

Muir, J. G., Rose, R., Rosella, O., Liels, K., Barrett, J. S., Shepherd, S. J., & Gibson, P. R. (2009). Measurement of short-chain carbohydrates in common Australian vegetables and fruits by high-performance liquid chromatography (HPLC). *Journal of Agricultural and Food Chemistry*, 57(2), 554-565.

Nanda, R., James, R., Smith, H., Dudley, C. R. K., & Jewell, D. P. (1989). Food intolerance and the irritable bowel syndrome. *Gut*, 30(8), 1099-1104.

National Digestive Diseases Information Clearinghouse (2014). Crohn's disease. *NIH Publication*, 14-3410.

National Digestive Diseases Information Clearinghouse (2014). Diverticular disease. *NIH Publication*, 13-1163.

National Digestive Diseases Information Clearinghouse (2014). Ulcerative colitis. *NIH Publication*, 14-1597.

Necas, J., Bartosikova, L. (2013). Carageenan: a review. *Veterinarni Medicina*, 58(4), 187-205.

Nelis, G. F., Vermeeren, M. A., & Jansen, W. (1990). Role of fruktose-sorbitol malabsorbtion in the irritable bowel syndrome. *Gastroenterology, 99*(4), 1016-1020.

Newburg, D. S. & Neubauer, S. H. (1995). Carbohydrates in milks: analysis, quantities, and significance. In Jensen, R. G. (Ed.), *Handbook of Milk Composition* (pp. 273-349). San Diego: Academic Press.

NICNAS (2008). Multiple chemical sensitivity: identifying key research needs. *Scientific Review Report.*

Nucera, G., Gabrielli, M., Lupascu, A., Lauritano, E. C., Santoliquido, A., cremonini, F., …Gasbarrini, A. (2005). Abnormal breath tests to laktose, fruktose and sorbitol in irritable bowel syndrome may be explained by small intestinal bacterial overgrowth. *Alimentary Pharmacology & Therapeutics, 21*(11), 1391-1395.

O'Connell, J. B., Maggard, M. A., & Ko, C. Y. (2004). Colon cancer survival rates with the new American Joint Committee on Cancer sixth edition staging. *Journal of the National Cancer Institute, 96*(19), 1420-1425.

O'Connell, S., & Walsh, G. (2006). Physicochemical characteristics of commercial lactases relevant to their application in the alleviation of laktose intolerance. *Applied Biochemistry and Biotechnology, 134*(2), 179-191.

Ong, D., Mitchell, S., Barrett, J., Shepherd, S., Irving, P., Biesiekierski, J., & … Muir, J. (2010). Manipulation of dietary short chain carbohydrates alters the pattern of gas production and genesis of symptoms in irritable bowel syndrome. *Journal of Gastroenterology & Hepatology, 25*(8), 1366-1373.

Park, Y. K., & Yetley, E. A. (1993). Intakes and food sources of fruktose in the United States. *The American Journal of Clinical Nutrition, 58*(5), 737S-747S.

Parker, T. J., Naylor, S. J., Riordan, A. M., & Hunter, J. O. (1995). Management of patients with food intolerance in irritable bowel syndrome. The development and use of an exclusion diet. *Journal of Human Nutrition and Dietetics, 8*(3), 159-166.

Peery, A. F., Barrett, P. R. Park, D., et al. (2012). A high-fiber diet does not protect against asymptomatic diverticulosis. *Gastroenterology, 142*(2), 266-272.

Petitpierre, M., Gumowski, P., & Girard, J. P. (1985). Irritable bowel syndrome and hypersensitivity to food. *Annals of Allergy, Asthma & Immunology, 54*(6), 538-540.

Quigley, E., Fried, M., Gwee, K. A., Olano, C., Guarner, F., Khalif, I., … & Le Mair, A. W. (2009). Irritable bowel syndrome: a global perspective. *WGO Practice Guideline.*

Quigley, E., M., M., Hunt, R. H., Emmanuel, A., & Hungin, A. P. S. (2013). *Irritable bowel syndrome (ibs): what is it, what causes it and can i do anything about it?* Retrieved from http://client.blueskybroadcastcom/WGO/ index.html.

Raithel, M., Weidenhiller, M., Hagel, A.-F.-K., Hetterich, U., Neurath, M. F., & Konturek, P. C. (2013). The malabsorption of commonly occurring mono and disaccharides: levels of investigation and differential diagnoses. *Dtsch Arztebl Int*, 110(46), 775-782.

Rex, D. K., Johnson, D. A., Anderson, J. C., Schoenfeld, P. S., Burke, C. A., & Inadomi, J. M. (2009). American College of Gastroenterology guidelines for colorectal cancer screening 2008. *The American Journal of Gastroenterology*, 104(3), 739-750.

Riby, J. E., Fujisawa, T., & Kretchmer, N. (1993). Fruktose absorption. *The American Journal of Clinical Nutrition*, 58(5), 748S-753S.

Ross, A. C., Manson, J. E., Abrams, S. A., Aloia, J. F., Brannon, P. M., Clinton, S. K., ... & Shapses, S. A. (2011). The 2011 report on dietary reference intakes for calcium and vitamin D from the Institute of Medicine: what clinicians need to know. *Journal of Clinical Endocrinology & Metabolism*, 96(1), 53-58.

Rubio-Tapia, A., Hill, I. D., Kelly, C. P., Calderwood, A. H., & Murray, J. A. (2013). ACG clinical guidelines: diagnosis and management of celiac disease.*The American Journal of Gastroenterology*, 108(5), 656-676.

Rumessen, J. J., & Gudmand-Høyer, E. (1986). Absorption capacity of fruktose in healthy adults. comparison with sucrose and its constituent monosaccharides. *Gut*, 27(10), 1161-1168.

Rumessen, J. J., & Gudmand-Høyer, E. (1987). Malabsoption of fruktose-sorbitol mixtures. Interactions causing abdominal distress. *Scandinavian Journal of Gastroenterology*, 22(4), 431-436.

Rumessen, J. J. (1992). Fruktose and related food carbohydrates. sources, intake, absorbtion, and clinical implications. *Scandinavian Journal of Gastroenterology*, 27(10), 819-828.

Ruppin, H., Bar-Meir, S., Soergel, K. H., Wood, C. M., & Schmitt Jr, M. G. (1980). Absorption of short-chain fatty acids by the colon. *Gastroenterology*, 78(6), 1500-1507.

Rycroft, C. E., Jones, M. R., Gibson, G. R., & Rastall, R. A. (2001). A comparative in vitro evaluation of the fermentation properties of prebiotic oligosaccharides. *Journal of Applied Microbiology*, 91(5), 878-887.

Scientific Community on Food (2000*). Opinion of the Scientific Committee on Food on the tolerable upper intake level of folate.* Retrieved from: www.ec.europa.eu/food/fc/sc/scf/out80e_en.pdf

Shepherd, S. J., & Gibson, P. R. (2006). Fruktose malabsorption and symptoms of irritable bowel syndrome: guidelines for effective dietary management. *Journal of the American Dietetic Association*, 106(10), 1631-1639.

Shepherd, S. J., Parker, F. C., Muir, J. G., & Gibson, P. R. (2008). Dietary triggers of abdominal symptoms in patients with irritable bowel syndrome: randomized placebo-controlled evidence. *Clinical Gastroenterology and Hepatology*, 6(7), 765-771.

Silk, D. B. A., Davis, A., Vulevic, J., Tzortzis, G., & Gibson, G. R. (2009). Clinical trial: the effects of a trans-galactooligosaccharide prebiotic on faecal microbiota and symptoms in irritable bowel syndrome. *Alimentary Pharmacology & Therapeutics*, 29(5), 508-518.

Simopoulos, A. P. (1999). Essential fatty acids in health and chronic disease. *The American Journal of Clinical Nutrition*, 70(3), 560s-569s.

Speier, C., Vessey, I., & Valacich, J. S. (2003). The effects of interruptions, task complexity, and information presentation on computer-supported decision-making performance. *Decision Sciences*, 34(4), 771-797.

Stefanini, G. F., Saggioro, A., Alvisi, V., Angelini, G., capurso, L., Di, L. G., …Melzi, G. (1995). Oral cromolyn sodium in comparison with elimination diet in the irritable bowel syndrome, diarrheic type. multicenter study of 428 patients. *Scandinavian Journal of Gastroenterology*, 30(6), 535–541.

Stockwell, M. (n. d.). *Awards/Events*. Retrieved from www.melissastock well.com/Melissa_Stockwell/Awards.html.

Stubbs, J. (2013). N. t.. In Wells, V., Wyness, L., & Coe, S. (Eds.). The British Nutrition Foundation's 45th anniversary conference: behaviour change in relation to healthier lifestyles. *Nutrition Bulletin*, 38(1), 100-107.

Suarez, F. L., Savaiano, D. A., & Levitt, M. D. (1995). A comparison of symptoms after the consumption of milk or lactose-hydrolyzed milk by people with self-reported severe lactose intolerance. *New England Journal of Medicine*, 333(1), 1-4.

Suarez, F. L., Springfield, J., Furne, J. K., Lohrmann, T. T., Kerr, P. S., & Levitt, M. D. (1999). Gas production in humans ingesting a soybean flour derived from beans naturally low in oligosaccharides. *The American Journal of Clinical Nutrition*, 69(1), 135-139.

Sundhedsstyrelsen og Fødevareministeriet (2009). *Cøliaki og mad uden Gluten* (4th ed.). København: Sundhedsstyrelsen.

Tarpila, S., Tarpila, A., Grohn, P., Silvennoinen, T., & Lindberg, L. (2004). Efficacy of ground flaxseed on constipation in patients with irritable bowel syndrome. *Current Topics in Nutraceutical Research*, 2(2), 119–125.

Test (2008). Schneller, schöner, stärker. *test – Journal Gesundheit*, 43(02), 88-92.

Teuri, U., Vapaatalo, H., & Korpela, R. (1999). Fructooligosaccharides and lactulose cause more symptoms in laktose maldigesters and subjects with pseudohypolactasia than in control laktose digesters. *The American Journal of Clinical Nutrition*, 69(5), 973-979.

Thompson, Kyle (2006). *Bristol Stool Chart* [Graphical illustration]. Retrieved from http://commons.wikimedia.org/wiki/File:Bristol_Stool_chart.png

Nanda, R., Shu, L. H., & Thomas, J. R. (2012). A fodmap diet update: craze or credible. *Practical Gastroenterology*, 10(12), 37-46.

Toschke, A. M., Thorsteinsdottir, K. H., & von Kries, R. (2009). Meal frequency, breakfast consumption and childhood obesity. *International Journal of Pediatric Obesity*, 4(4), 242-248.

Tou, J. C., Chen, J., & Thompson, L. U. (1998). Flaxseed and its lignan precursor, secoisolariciresinol diglycoside, affect pregnancy outcome and reproductive development in rats. *The Journal of Nutrition*, 128(11), 1861-1868.

Truswell, A. S., Seach, J. M., & Thorburn, A. W. (1988). Incomplete absorption of pure fruktose in healthy subjects and the facilitating effect of glucose. *The American Journal of Clinical Nutrition*, 48(6), 1424-1430.

U. S. Department of Agriculture and U. S. Department of Health and Human Services (2010). *Dietary Guidelines for Americans* (7th ed.). Washington, Dc: U. S. Government Printing Office.

U. S. Department of Agriculture, Agricultural Research Service (2013). *USDA National Nutrient Database for Standard Reference*, Release 26. Retrieved from: http://www.ars.usda.gov/ba/bhnrc /ndl.

van Loo, J., Coussement, P., De Leenheer, L., Hoebregs, H., & Smits, G. (1995). On the presence of inulin and oligofruktose as natural ingredients in the western diet. *Critical Reviews in Food Science and Nutrition*, 35(6), 525–552.

Varea, V., de Carpi, J. M., Puig, C., Alda, J. A., camacho, E., Ormazabal, A., ... & Gómez, L. (2005). Malabsorption of carbohydrates and depression in Children and adolescents. *Journal of Pediatric Gastroenterology and Nutrition*, 40(5), 561-565.

Verhoef, P., Stampfer, M. J., Buring, J. F., Gaziano, J. M., Allen, R. H., Stabler, S. P., ... & Willett, W. C. (1996). Homocysteine metabolism and risk of myocardial infarction: relation with vitamins B6, B12, and folate. *American Journal of Epidemiology*, 143(9), 845-859.

Vernia, P., Ricciardi, M. R., Frandina, C., Bilotta, T., & Frieri, G. (1995). laktose malabsorption and irritable bowel syndrome. Effect of a long-term laktose-free diet. *The Italian Journal of Gastroenterology*, 27(3), 117-121.

Vesa, T. H., Korpela, R. A., & Sahi, T. (1996). Tolerance to small amounts of laktose in laktose maldigesters. *The AmericanJournal of Clinical Nutrition*, 64(2), 197-20.

Virtanen, S. M., Räsänen, L., Mäenpää, J., & Åkerblom, H. K. (1987). Dietary survey of Finnish adolescent diabetics and non-diabetic controls. *Acta Paediatrica*, 76(5), 801-808.

Vos, M. B., Kimmons, J. E., Gillespie, C., Welsh, J., & Blanck, H. M. (2008). Dietary fruktose consumption among US children and adults: the third National Health and Nutrition Examination Survey. *The Medscape Journal of Medicine*, 10(7), 160.

Watson, B. D. (2008). Public health and carrageenan regulation : a review and analysis. *Journal of Applied Phycology*, 20(5), 505-513.

Webb, F. S., & Whitney, E. N. (2008). *Nutrition: Concepts and Controversies* (11th ed.). Belmont, CA: Thomson/ Wadsworth.

Wedlake, L., Slack, N., Andreyev, H. J. N., & Whelan, K. (2014). Fiber in the treatment and maintenance of inflammatory bowel disease: a systematic review of randomized controlled trials. *Inflammatory bowel diseases*, 20(3), 576-586.

Welch, C. E., Allen, A. W., & Donaldons, G. A. (1953). An appraisal of resection of the colon for diverticulitis of the sigmoid. *Annals of Surgery*, 138(3), 332-343.

Wells, N. E. J., Hahn, B. A., & Whorwell, P. J. (1997). Clinical economics review: irritable bowel syndrome. *Allimentary Pharmacology and Therapeutics*, 11, 1019-1030.

—

Sources regarding the prevalence of IBS:
USA

Longstreth, G. F., & Wolde-Tsadik, G. (1993). Irritable bowel-type symptoms in hmo examinees. *Digestive Diseases and Sciences*, 38(9), 1581-1589.

Talley, N. J., Zinsmeister, A. R., van Dyke, C., & Melton, L. J. (1991). Epidemiology of colonic symptoms and the irritable bowel syndrome. *Gastroenterology*, 101(4), 927-934.

O'Keefe, E. A., Talley, N. J., Zinsmeister, A. R., & Jacobsen, S. J. (1995). Bowel disorders impair functional status and quality of life in the elerdly: a population-based study. *Journal of Gastroenterology*, 50A, M184-M189.

Great Britain

Jones, R., & Lydeard, S. (1992). Irritable bowel syndrom in the general population. *British Medical Journal*, 304(6819), 87-90.

Japan and the Netherlands

Schlemper, R. J., van der Werf, S. D. J., Vandenbroucke, J. P., Blemond, I., & Lamers, C. B. H. W. (1993). Peptic ulcer, non-ulcer dysepsia and irritable bowel syndrom in the Netherlands and Japan. *Scandinavian Journal of Gastroenterology*, 28(200), 33-41.

Nigeria

Olubuykle, I. O., Olawuyl, F., & Fasanmade, A. A. (1995). A study of irritable bowel syndrom diagnosed by manning Criteria in an African population. *Digestive Diseases and Sciences*, 40(5), 983-985.

—

Wilder-Smith, C. H., Materna, A., Wermelinger, C., & Schuler, J. (2013). Fruktose and laktose intolerance and malabsorption testing: the relationship with symptoms in functional gastrointestinal disorders. *Alimentary Pharmacology and Therapeutics*, 37(11), 1074-1083.

Winterfeldt, D. von, & Edwards, W. (1986). *Decision Analysis and Behavioral Research*. Cambridge: Cambridge University Press.

Wittstock, A. (1949). *Marc Aurel – Selbstbetrachtungen*. Stuttgart: Reclam.

Zohar, D. (1999). When things go wrong: The effect of daily work hassles on effort, exertion and negative mood. *Journal of Occupational and Organizational Psychology*, 72(3), 265-283.

Food Index

A

3 Musketeers® 134

7 UP® 110

9-grain Wheat bread 155

After Eight® Thin Chocolate Mints 134

Ale 97

Alfalfa sprouts 164

All-Bran® Original (Kellogg's®) 114

Almond butter, salted 117

Almond butter, unsalted 117

Almond cookies 129

Almond milk, vanilla or other flavors, unsweetened 121

Almond paste (Marzipan) 134

Almonds, honey roasted 134

Almonds, raw 126

Alpine Lace 25% Reduced Fat, Mozzarella 117

Amaranth Flakes (Arrowhead Mills) 114

Amaretto 97

American cheese 155

American cheese, processed 117

Americano, decaf, without flavored syrup 103

Americano, with flavored syrup 103

Americano, without flavored syrup 103

Apple banana strawberry juice 107

Apple cake, glazed 129

Apple grape juice 107

Apple juice or cider, made from frozen 97

Apple juice or cider, unsweetened 97

Apple strudel 129

Applejack liquor 97

Applesauce, canned, sweetened 159

Applesauce, canned, unsweetened 159

Apricot nectar 107

Apricot, dried, cooked, sweetened 159

Apricot, dried, uncooked 159

Apricot, fresh 159

Aquavit 97

Arby's® macaroni and cheese 139

Arby's® orange juice 107

Archway® Ginger Snaps 129

Archway® Oatmeal Raisin Cookies 129

Archway® Peanut Butter Cookies 129

Artichoke, globe raw 164

Arugula, raw 164

Asian noodle bowl, vegetables only 139

Asparagus, raw 164

Au gratin potato, prepared from fresh 148

Avocado, green skin, Florida type 164

B

Baby food, Gerber Graduates® Organic Pasta Pick-Ups Three Cheese Ravioli 139

Baby food, zwieback 126

bacon 155

Bacon EGG® and Cheese BK Muffin® 150

Baguette 112

Baking powder 174

Bamboo shoots, canned and drained 164

Banana, chips 159

Banana, fresh 159

Barbecue sauce 150

Barley flour 174

Basmati rice, cooked in unsalted water 148

BBQ roasted jalapeno sauce 150

Beef bacon (kosher) 144

Beef steak, chuck, visible fat eaten 144

Beef with noodles soup, condensed 139

Beer 97

Beer, low alcohol 97

Beer, low carb 97

Beer, non alcoholic 97

Beets, raw 164

Ben & Jerry's® Ice Cream, Brownie Batter 171

Ben & Jerry's® Ice Cream, Chocolate Chip Cookie Dough 171

Ben & Jerry's® Ice Cream, Chubby Hubby® 171

Ben & Jerry's® Ice Cream, Chunky Monkey® 171

Ben & Jerry's® Ice Cream, Half Baked 171

Ben & Jerry's® Ice Cream, Karamel Sutra® 171

Ben & Jerry's® Ice Cream, New York Super Fudge Chunk® 171

Ben & Jerry's® Ice Cream, One Sweet Whirled 171

Ben & Jerry's® Ice Cream, Peanut Butter Cup 171

Ben & Jerry's® Ice Cream, Phish Food® 171

Ben & Jerry's® Ice Cream, Vanilla For A Change 171

Biscotti, chocolate, nuts 129

BK Big Fish® 150

BK Fresh Apple Slices 150

Black beans, cooked from dried 164

Black cherry juice 107

Black currant juice 107

Black olives 164

Black Russian 97

Blackberries, fresh 159

Blackberry juice 107

Bloody Mary 97

BLT Salad® with TenderCrisp chicken (no dressing or croutons) 150

Blue cheese 117

Blueberries, fresh 159

Bockwurst 144

Bok choy, raw 164

Bologna, beef ring 117

Bologna, combination of meats, light (reduced fat) 117

Boston Market® 1/4 white rotisserie chicken, with skin 144

Boston Market® macaroni and cheese 139

Boston Market® roasted turkey breast 144

Boston Market® sweet corn 148

Bourbon 97

Boysenberries, fresh 159

Brandy 97

Bratwurst 144

Bratwurst, beef 144

Bratwurst, light (reduced fat) 144

Bratwurst, made with beer 144

Bratwurst, made with beer, cheese-filled 144

Bratwurst, turkey 144

Braunschweiger 144

Brazil nuts, unsalted 126

Breath mint, regular 134

Breath mint, sugar free 134

Breyers® Ice Cream, Natural Vanilla, Lactose Free 171

Breyers® Light! Boosts Immunity Yogurt, all flavors 121

Breyers® No Sugar Added Ice Cream, Vanilla 121

Breyers® YoCrunch Light Nonfat Yogurt, with granola 121

Brie cheese 117
Broccoli flower (green cauliflower), cooked 164
Broccoli, raw 164
Brown mushrooms (Italian or Crimini, raw 164
Brown sugar 134
Brownie, chocolate, fat free 129
Brussels sprouts, cooked from fresh 164
Bulgur, home cooked 148
Burgundy wine, red 98
Burgundy wine, white 98
Butter cracker 129
Butter, light, salted 117
Butter, unsalted 117
Buttermels® (Switzer's®) 134
Butternut squash soup 139

C
Cabbage, green, cooked 165
Cabbage, red, cooked 165
Cabbage, savoy, raw 165

Cabot® Non Fat Yogurt, plain 121
Cabot® Non Fat Yogurt, vanilla 121
Caesar Salad (no dressing or croutons) 150
Caesar salad dressing 152
Cafe au lait, without flavored syrup 103
Cafe latte, flavored syrup 103
Cafe latte, without flavored syrup 103
Calzone, cheese 139
Camembert cheese 117
Camomile tea 103
Campari® 98
Candy necklace 134
Canfield's® Root Beer 110
Canfield's® Root Beer, diet 110
Cantaloupe, fresh 159
Cape Cod 98
Cappuccino, canned 103
Cappuccino, decaf, with flavored syrup 103

Cappuccino, decaf, without flavored syrup 103
Capri Sun®, all flavors 107
Carambola (starfruit), fresh 159
Caramel or sugar coated popcorn, store bought 126
Carrot cake, glazed, homemade 129
Carrot juice 107
Carrots, cooked from fresh 165
Carrots, raw 165
Cascadian Farm® Organic Gran. Bar, Dark Chocolate Cranberry 114
Cashews, raw 126
Casserole (hot dish), with tomato 147
Casserole (hot dish), rice with beef, tomato base, vegetables other than dark green, cheese or gravy 139
Cauliflower, cooked from frozen 165
Caviar 144

Celeriac (celery root), cooked from fresh 165
Celery, cooked 165
Chai tea 103
Chalupas Supreme® with beef, beans, cheese 157
Champagne punch 98
Champagne, white 98
Chard, raw or blanched, marinated in oil 165
Chardonnay 98
Chayote squash, cooked 165
Cheddar cheese 155
Cheddar cheese, natural 117
Cheerios® Snack Mix, all 114
Cheese cracker 126
Cheese gnocchi 148
Cheese sauce, store bought 117
Cheeseburger 150
Cheesecake, plain or flavored, homemade 129
Cherry Coke® 110

Cherry pie, bottom crust only 129
Chestnuts, boiled, steamed 165
Chestnuts, roasted 126
Chewing gum 134
Chewing gum, sugar free 134
Chia seeds 126
Chicken and dumplings soup, condensed 139
Chicken breast, spicy crispy 152
Chicken cake or patty 147
Chicken fricassee with gravy, American style 144
Chicken Littles with sauce 152
Chicken noodle soup with vegetables, can 139
Chicken with cheese sauce, vegetables other than dark green 147
Chicken wonton soup, prepared from condensed can 139

Chicory coffee 103
Chicory coffee powder, unprepared 165
Chicory greens, raw 165
Chili with beans, beef, canned 139
Chipotle southwest salad dressing 155
Chips Ahoy!® Chewy Gooey Caramel Cookies (Nabisco®) 129
Chobani® Nonfat Greek Yogurt, Black Cherry 121
Chobani® Nonfat Greek Yogurt, Lemon 121
Chobani® Nonfat Greek Yogurt, Peach 121
Chobani® Nonfat Greek Yogurt, Raspberry 121
Chobani® Nonfat Greek Yogurt, Strawberry 121
Chocolate cake, glazed, store 129
Chocolate Chex® (General Mills®) 114
Chocolate chip cookie 155

Chocolate chip cookies, store bought 130
Chocolate chunk cookie 155
Chocolate cookies, iced, store bought 130
Chocolate pudding, store bought 121
Chocolate pudding, store bought, no sugar 121
Chocolate sandwich cookies, double filling 130
Chocolate sandwich cookies, sugar free 130
Chocolate truffles 134
Chop suey, chicken 140
Chop suey, tofu, no noodles 140
Cinnamon crispas 130
Cinnamon toast crunch® (General Mills®) 114
Cinnamon Toasters® (Malt-O-Meal®) 114
Clams, with mushroom, onions, & bread 144

Classic Fruit Chocolates (Liberty Orchards®) 134
Clementine, fresh 159
Clif Bar®,Chocolate Chip 95
Clif Bar®,Crunchy Peanut Butter 95
Clif Bar®,Oatmeal Raisin Walnut 95
Club soda 98
Cocoa Krispies® (Kellogg's®) 114
Cocoa Puffs® (General Mills®) 114
Coconut Bars, nuts 134
Coconut cream (liquid from grated meat) 126
Coconut milk, fresh (liquid from grated meat, water added) 126
Coconut, dried, shredded or flaked, unsweetened 126
Coconut, fresh 126
Coffee substitute, prepared 103

Coffee, prepared from flavored mix, no sugar 103
Cognac 98
Cointreau® 98
Coke Zero® 110
Coke® 110
Coke® with Lime 110
Colby Jack cheese 117
Cole slaw 152
Coleslaw, with apples and raisins, mayo dressing 165
Coleslaw, with pineapple, mayo dressing 165
Collards, raw 165
Corn Chex® (General Mills®) 114
Corn Flakes (Kellogg's®) 114
Cornbread, from mix 148
Cornbread, homemade 148
Cottage cheese, 1% fat, lactose reduced 117
Cottage cheese, uncreamed dry curd 121
Couscous, cooked 148

Cracked wheat bread, with raisins 112
Cranberries, dried (Craisins®) 160
Cranberries, fresh 160
Cranberry juice cocktail, with apple juice 107
Cranberry juice cocktail, with blueberry juice 107
Cream cheese spread 118
Cream cheese, whipped, flavored 118
Cream cheese, whipped, plain 118
Cream of asparagus soup, condensed can 140
Cream of broccoli soup, condensed 140
Cream of celery soup, homemade 140
Cream of chicken soup, condensed 140
Cream of mushroom soup, from condensed can 140

Cream of potato soup mix, dry 140
Cream of spinach soup mix, dry 140
Creamed chicken 147
Creamy buffalo sauce 152
Creme de Cocoa 98
Creme de menthe 98
Crepe, plain 130
Crispy Chicken Caesar Salad 152
Crispy Twister without sauce 152
Crispy Twister® with sauce 152
Croissant, chocolate 130
Croissant, fruit 130
Crunchy Nut Roasted Nut & Honey (Kellogg's®) 114
Cucumber, raw, with peel 166

Cucumber, raw, without peel 166
Curacao 98
Currants, fresh, black 160
Currants, fresh, red and white 160

D

Daiquiri 98
Dairy Queen® Foot Long Hot Dog 140
Dandelion tea 104
Danish pastry, frosted, with cheese filling 130
Dannon® Activia® Light Yogurt, vanilla 122
Dannon® Activia® Yogurt, plain 122
Dannon® Greek Yogurt Honey 122
Dannon® Greek Yogurt, Plain 122
Dannon® la Crème Yogurt, fruit flavors 122
Dare Breaktime Ginger Cookies 130
Dare® Lemon Crème Cookies 130
Dark chocolate Bar 50% 134
Dark chocolate Bar 60%-69% cacao 135
Dark chocolate Bar 70%-85% cacao 135

Dark chocolate Bar, sugar free 135

Dark Fruit Chocolates (Liberty Orchards®) 135

Dark Fruit Chocolates, Sugar Free (Liberty Orchards®) 135

Dates 160

Demitasse 104

Diet 7 UP® 110

Diet Coke® 110

Diet Dr. Pepper® 110

Diet Pepsi®, fountain 110

Doritos® Tortilla Chips, Nacho Cheese 126

Doughnut, glazed, coconut topping 130

Doughnut, glazed, plain 130

Doughnut, sugared 130

Dove® Promises, Milk Chocolate 104

Dreyer's® Grand Ice Cream, Chocolate 171

Dreyer's® No Sugar Added Ice Cream, Triple Chocolate 171

Drumstick® (sundae cone) 172

E

Earl Grey, strong 104

Edam cheese 118

EGG® bread roll 130

Eggnog, regular 98

Eggplant, cooked 166

Elderberries, fresh 160

Electrolyte drink 95

Elephant ear (crispy) 130

Endive, curly, raw 166

English muffin bread 112

English muffin, whole wheat, with raisins 131

Enoki mushrooms, raw 166

Espresso, raw 104

Essentials Oat Bran cereal (Quaker®) 114

Evaporated milk, diluted, 2% fat (reduced fat) 122

Evaporated milk, skim (fat free) 104

Evaporated milk, whole 122

Extra Crispy Tenders 152

F

Falafel 148

Familia Swiss Muesli® 114

Fanta Zero®, fruit flavors 110

Fanta® Red 110

Fanta®, fruit flavors 110

Fennel bulb 166

Fennel tea 104

Feta cheese 122

Feta cheese, fat free 122

Fettuccini Alfredo®, no meat, carrots or dark green veggies 140

Fettuccini Alfredo®, no meat, vegetables except dark green 140

Fettuccini noodles 148

Fiber One Original® (General Mills®) 115

Fiber One® Nutty Clusters & Almonds (General Mills®) 115

Fifty 50® Sugar Free Butterscotch Hard Candy 135

Figs, dried, cooked, sweetened 160

Figs, fresh 160

Filberts, raw 126

Fish croquette 147

Fish or seafood with cream or white sauce 147

Fish sticks, patties / nuggets, breaded, 145

Fish with breading 145

Flax seeds, not fortified 126

Fleischmann's® Butter Margarine, tub, whipped 118

Focaccia bread 112

Fondue sauce 122

Frappuccino® 104

Frappuccino®, bottled or canned 104

Frappuccino®, bottled light 104

French Burnt Peanuts 135

French fries 150

French or Vienna roll 112

French toast 131

Froot Loops® (Kellogg's®) 115

Frosted Flakes®
(Kellogg's®) 115
Frosted Flakes®
Reduced Sugar
(Kellogg's®) 115
Frosted Mini-
Wheats Big Bite®
(Kellogg's®) 115
Frozen custard,
chocolate or cof-
fee flavors 131
Frozen fruit juice
Bar 172
Fruit drink or
punch 107
Fruit punch, alco-
holic 98
Fruit sauce, jelly-
based 140

G
Garbanzo beans
canned 148
Garlic, fresh 166
Gatorade®, all fla-
vors 95
Gelatin, jello 135
German choco-
late cake, glazed,
homemade 131
German style po-
tato salad, with
bacon and vine-
gar dressing 140
GG® Scandina-
vian Bran Crisp-
bread 112

Gibson 99
Gin 99
Ginger ale 110
Ginger root, raw
166
Ginko nuts, dried
127
Girl Scout® Lem-
onades 131
Girl Scout® Pea-
nut Butter Patties
131
Girl Scout® Sa-
moas® 131
Girl Scout® Short-
bread® 131
Girl Scout® Thin
Mints 131
Glaceau® Vita-
minwater 95
Gluten free bread
112
GO Veggie!™
Rice Slices 122
Goat cheese, hard
118
GoLEAN® Crisp!
Cereal, Cinna-
mon Crumble
(Kashi®) 115
GoLEAN®
Crunch! Cereal,
Honey Almond
Flax (Kashi®) 115
Gooseberries,
fresh 160
Gorgonzola
cheese 118

Gorton's® Bat-
tered Fish Fillets
145
Gorton's® Pop-
corn Shrimp,
Original 145
Gouda cheese 118
Goulash, with
beef, noodles, to-
mato base 145
Grand Marnier®
99
Grapefruit juice,
white 107
Grapefruit, fresh,
pink or red 160
Grapes, fresh 160
Grasshopper 99
Greek yogurt,
plain, nonfat, 122
Green beans
(string beans),
cooked 166
Green bell pep-
pers 166
Green olives 166
Green pea soup
140
Green peas, raw
148
Green tea, strong
104
Green tomato,
raw 166
Grits (polenta)
166
Guava (guayaba),
fresh, 160

Gum drops 135
Gum drops,
sugar free 135
Gummi bears 135
Gummi bears,
sugar free 135
Gummi dino-
saurs 135
Gummi dino-
saurs, no sugar
135
Gummi worms
135
Gummi worms,
sugar free 136

H
Haagen-Dazs®
Creme Brulee 172
Haagen-Dazs®
Frozen Yogurt,
chocolate or cof-
fee flavors 172
Haagen-Dazs®
Frozen Yogurt,
vanilla or other
flavors 172
Haagen-Dazs® Ice
Cream, Bailey's
Irish Cream 172
Haagen-Dazs® Ice
Cream, Black
Walnut 172
Haagen-Dazs® Ice
Cream, Butter Pe-
can 172

Haagen-Dazs® Cherry Vanilla 172

Haagen-Dazs® Ice Cream, Chocolate 172

Haagen-Dazs® Ice Cream, Coffee 172

Haagen-Dazs® Ice Cream, Cookies & Cream 172

Haagen-Dazs® Ice Cream, Mango 172

Haagen-Dazs® Ice Cream, Pistachio 172

Haagen-Dazs® Ice Cream, Rocky Road 172

Haagen-Dazs® Ice Cream, Strawberry 173

Haagen-Dazs® Ice Cream, Vanilla Chocolate Chip 173

Half and half 122

Halvah 131

Ham croquette 147

Ham Sandwich with Veggies, no mayo 155

Hamburger 150

Hard candy 136

Hard candy, sugar free 136

Hardee's® Loaded Omelet Biscuit 140

Harvey Wall-banger 99

Health Valley® Multigrain Chewy Granola Bar, Chocolate Chip 115

Herbal tea 104

Herring, pickled 145

Hershey's® Bliss Hot Drink White Chocolate, prepared 104

Hershey's® Caramel Filled Chocolates no sugar 136

Hershey's® Milk Chocolate Bar 136

Hickorynuts 127

High-protein Bar, generic 95

Honey 115

Honey BBQ sauce 152

Honey mustard dressing 155

Honey Nut Chex® (General Mills®) 115

Honey Oat bread 155

Honey Smacks® (Kellogg's®) 115

Honeydew 160

Hot chili peppers, green, cooked 166

Hot chili peppers, red, cooked from fresh 166

Hot chocolate, homemade 104

Hot dog, combination of meats, plain 118

Hot wings 152

House side salad 152

Hubbard squash 167

I

Ice cream sandwich 173

Ice cream, light 173

Instant coffee mix, unprepared 104

Irish coffee with alcohol and whipped cream 104

Italian BMT® Sandwich with Veggies, no mayo 155

J

Jackfruit, fresh 160

Jam 118

Jam no sugar or sweetener 119

Jasmine tea 105

Jelly beans® 136

Jelly beans®, sugar free 136

Jerusalem artichoke raw 167

Jujyfruits® 136

K

Kale, raw 167

Kamikaze 99

Kashi® Chewy Granola Bar, Cherry Dark Chocolate 115

Kashi® Layered Granola Bar, Pumpkin Pecan 136

Kefir 122

Kelp, raw 167

Ken's® Apple Cider Vinaigrette dressing 150

Kern's® Mango-Orange Nectar 107

Kern's® Strawberry Nectar 107

Kidney beans, cooked from dried 167

Kirsch 99

Kit Kat® 136

Kit Kat® White 136

Kiwi fruit, gold 160

Kiwi fruit, green 160

Kohlrabi, cooked 167

Kraft® Cheese Spread, Roka Blue 119

L

Lasagna, home-made, beef 141

Lasagna, home-made, cheese, no vegetables 141

Lasagna, home-made, spinach, no meat 141

Laughing Cow® Mini Babybel®, Cheddar 122

Laughing Cow® Mini Babybel®, Original 123

Lay's® Potato Chips 127

Lay's® Potato Chips, Sour Cream & Onion 127

Lay's® Stax Potato Crisps, Cheddar 127

Lay's® Stax Potato Crisps, Hot 'n Spicy 127

Lebkuchen (German ginger bread) 131

Leeks, leafs 167

Leeks, root 167

Leeks, whole 167

Lemon juice, fresh 108

Lemon peel 174

Lemon, fresh 161

Lentil soup, condensed 141

Lentils, cooked from dried 148

Lettuce, Boston, bibb or butterhead 167

Lettuce, green leaf 167

Lettuce, iceberg 167

Lettuce, red leaf 167

Lettuce, romaine or cos 167

Libby's® Apricot Nectar 108

Libby's® Banana Nectar 108

Libby's® Juicy Juice®, Apple Grape 108

Libby's® Juicy Juice®, Grape 108

Libby's® Pear Nectar 108

Licorice 136

Licuado, mango 123

Light beer 99

Light cream 123

Lima beans, cooked from dried 167

Limburger cheese 119

Lime juice, fresh 108

Lime, fresh 161

Lipton® Iced Tea Mix, sweetened with sugar, prepared 196

Lipton® Instant 100% Tea, unsweetened, prepared 196

Liqueur, coffee flavored 99

Little Debbie® Coffee Cake, Apple Streusel 131

Little Debbie® Fudge Brownies with Walnuts 131

Little Debbie® Nutty Bars 136

Liver pudding 145

Loaf cold cut, spiced 147

Loganberries, fresh 161

Long Island iced tea 99

Long John or bismarck, glazed, cream or custard filled & nuts 131

Lotus root, cooked 168

Lowbush cranberries (lingonberries) 161

Lychees (litchis), fresh 161

Lycium (wolf or goji berries) 161

Lyonnaise (potatoes and onions) 141

M & M® cookie 155

M & M's® Peanut 136

Macadamia nuts, raw 127

Macaroni or pasta salad, with meat, egg, mayo dressing 141

Mai Tai 99

Maitake mushrooms, raw 168

Malt liquor 99

Mamba® Fruit Chews 136

Mamba® Sour Fruit Chews 136

M

Mandarin orange, fresh 161

Mango nectar 108

Mango, fresh 161
Mangosteen, fresh 161
Manhattan 99
Maple syrup, pure 115
Margarine, diet, fat free 119
Margarine, tub, salted, sunflower oil 119
Margarita, frozen 99
Marmalade, sugar free with aspartame 119
Marmalade with saccharin 119
Marmalade, sugar free with sucralose 119
Marshmallow 137
Martini® 99
Mascarpone 119
Mashed potatoes with gravy 152
McDonald's® apple slices 153
McDonald's® Barbecue sauce 153
McDonald's® Big Mac® 153
McDonald's® caramel sundae® 153
McDonald's® Cheeseburger 153

McDonald's® Chicken McNuggets® 153
McDonald's® chocolate chip cookies 153
McDonald's® chocolate milk 153
McDonald's® Crispy Chicken Snack Wrap with ranch sauce 153
McDonald's® Double Cheeseburger 153
McDonald's® Filet-O-Fish® 153
McDonald's® French fries 153
McDonald's® Hamburger 153
McDonald's® hot fudge sundae® 153
McDonald's® hot mustard 153
McDonald's® M & M McFlurry® 154
McDonald's® McCafe shakes, chocolate 154
McDonald's® McCafe shakes, vanilla or other flavors 154

McDonald's® McChicken® 154
McDonald's® McDouble® 154
McDonald's® McRib® 154
McDonald's® Newman's Own® Creamy Caesar dressing 154
McDonald's® Newman's Own® Low Fat Balsamic Vinaigrette salad dressing 154
McDonald's® orange juice 154
McDonald's® Quarter Pounder 154
McDonald's® Sausage & EGG® McMuffin® 154
McDonald's® side salad 154
McDonald's® smoothies, all flavors 154
McDonald's® Southwestern chipotle Barbecue sauce 154
McDonald's® sweet and sour sauce 154
Meat ravioli, with tomato sauce 141

Meatloaf, pork 147
Meatloaf, tuna 147
Melba Toast®, Classic (Old London®) 127
Mentos® 137
Merlot, red 99
Merlot, white 100
Milk chocolate Bar, cereal 137
Milk chocolate Bar, cereal, sugar free 137
Milk chocolate Bar, sugar free 137
Milk Chocolate covered raisins 137
Milk Maid® Caramels (Brach's®) 137
Milk, low lactose Lactaid®, skim (fat free) 123
Milk, lactose reduced Lactaid®, fortified 115
Milk, low lactose Lactaid® 105
Milk, unprepared dry powder, 105
Mineral Water 196
Minestrone soup, condensed 141

Minestrone soup, homemade 141
Mint Julep 100
Mocha, pure 105
Mojito 100
Molasses cookies, store bought 131
Molasses, dark 137
Monster® Energy® 196
Monster® Khaos 196
Morel mushrooms, raw 168
Mortadella 119
Mountain Dew® 196
Mountain Dew® Code Red 196
Mozzarella, fat free 123
Mrs. Paul's® Calamari Rings 145
Muenster cheese, natural 119
Mueslix® (Kellogg's®) 116
Muffins, banana 131
Muffins, blueberry 132
Muffins, carrot, homemade, with nuts 132
Muffins, store bought 132

Muffins, pumpkin, 132
Mulberries 161
Mung bean sprouts 168
Mung beans, cooked from dried 168
Murray® Sugar Free Oatmeal Cookies 132
Murray® Sugar Free Shortbread 132
Muscatel 100
Mushrooms, batter dipped or breaded 168
Muskmelon 161
Mustard 155

N
Nabisco® 100 Calorie Packs, Honey Maid Cinnamon Roll 132
Nectarine 161
Nestea® 100% Tea, dry 196
Nestea® Iced Tea, Sugar Free, dry 196
Nestea® Iced Tea, no sugar 196Nestea® Iced Tea, with sugar, dry 196

Nestle® Hot Cocoa Dark Chocolate, prepared 105
Nestle® Hot Cocoa Rich Milk Chocolate 105
Nestle® Nesquik®, chocolate dry 137
Newman's Own® Organic Pretzels 112
Nilla Wafers® (Nabisco®) 132
No Fear® 196
No Fear® Sugar Free 196
Non-alcoholic wine 100
Noodle soup mix, dry 141
Northland® Cranberry Juice, all flavors 108
Nougat 137
Nutella® (filbert spread) 119
Nutter Butter® Cookies (Nabisco®) 132

O
Oat milk 123
Oatmeal cookies, store bought 132
Okra, raw 168
Old Dutch® Crunch Curls 127

Omelet, made with bacon 141
Omelet, made with sausage, potatoes, onions, cheese 141
Onion rings 150
Onion, white, yellow or red, raw 168
Oolong tea 105
Orange kiwi passion juice 108
Orange peel 174
Orange, fresh 161
Oreo® Brownie Cookies 132
Oreo® Cookies (Nabisco®) 132
Oreo® Cookies, Sugar Free 132
Chicken Crisp® Sandwich 150
Ouzo 100
Oven Roasted Chicken Sandwich with Veggies, no mayo 155
Oyster mushrooms, raw 168

P
Pad Thai, without meat 141
Paella 141
Pancake, buckwheat 132

Pancake, whole wheat, homemade 132

Pancakes and syrup 151

Panda Express® Orange Chicken 141

Papaya, fresh 161

Parmesan cheese, dry (grated) 123

Parmesan cheese, dry (grated), non-fat 123

Parmesan Oregano bread 155

Parsnip, cooked 168

Passion fruit (maracuya), fresh 161

Passion fruit juice 108

Pasta salad with vegetables, Italian dressing 141

Peach juice 108

Peach pie, bottom crust only 132

Peach, fresh 161

Peanut butter, unsalted 127

Peanuts, dry roasted, salted 127

Pear juice 108

Pear, fresh 162

Pecan praline 137

Pepperidge Farm® Soft Sugar Cookies 133

Pepperidge Farm® Turnover, Apple 133

Pepsi® 196

Pepsi® Max 196

Pepsi® Twist 196

Persimmon, fresh 162

Pho soup (Vietnamese soup) 142

Picante taco sauce 151

Pickled beef 145

Pickled beets 168

Pillsbury® Big White Chunk Macadamia Nut Cookies 133

Pillsbury® Cinnamon Roll with Icing, all flavors 133

Pina colada 100

Pine nuts, pignolias 127

Pineapple juice 108

Pineapple orange drink 108

Pineapple, dried 162

Pineapple, fresh 162

Pistachio nuts, raw 127

Pizza Hut® cheese bread stick 142

Pizza Hut® Pepperoni Lover's pizza, stuffed crust 142

Pizza Hut® Personal Pan, supreme 142

Pizza, homemade or restaurant, cheese, thin crust 142

Plain dumplings for stew, biscuit type 148

Plantains, green, boiled 162

Plum, fresh 162

Polenta 149

Pomegranate juice 108

Pomegranate, fresh (arils-seed/juice sacs) 162

Poore Brothers® Potato Chips, Salt & Cracked Pepper 127

Popcorn, store bought (prepopped), "buttered" 133

Popsicle 173

Popsicle, sugar free 173

Pork cutlet, visible fat eaten 145

Port wine 100

Portabella mushrooms 168

Potato bread 112

Potato chips, salted 127

Potato dumpling (Kartoffelkloesse) 149

Potato gnocchi 149

Potato pancakes 149

Potato salad, with egg, mayo dressing 142

Potato soup with broccoli and cheese 142

Potato sticks 128

Potato, boiled, with skin 149

Potato, boiled, without skin 149

Power Bar® 20g Protein Plus, Chocolate Crisp 95

Power Bar® 20g Protein Plus, Chocolate Peanut Butter 95

Power Bar® 30g Protein Plus, Chocolate Brownie 96

Power Bar® Harvest Energy®, Double Chocolate Crisp 96

Power Bar® Performance Energy® 96

Powerade®, all flavors 96

Pretzels, hard, unsalted, sticks 128

Pringles® Light Fat Free Potato Crisps, Barbecue 128

Pringles® Potato Crisps, Loaded Baked Potato 128

Pringles® Potato Crisps, Original 128

Pringles® Potato Crisps, Salt & Vinegar 128

Pudding mix, other flavors, cooked type 123

Pumpernickel roll 112

Pumpkin or squash seeds 128

Purslane, raw 168

Q

Quince, fresh 162

Quinoa 149

R

Radicchio, raw 168

Radish, raw 168

Raisins, uncooked 162

Rambutan, canned in syrup 162

Ranch Crispy Chicken Wrap 151

Ranch salad dressing 156

Raspberries, fresh, red 162

Raspberry juice 109

Ratatouille 142

Red beans and rice soup mix, dry 142

Red Bull® Energy Drink 111

Red Bull® Energy Drink Sugar Free 111

Rhubarb pie, bottom crust only 133

Rhubarb, fresh 162

Ribs, beef, spare, visible fat eaten 145

Rice bread 112

Rice cake 128

Rice Krispies® (Kellogg's®) 116

Rice milk 123

Rice noodles, fried 149

Rice pudding (arroz con leche), coconut, raisins 123

Rice pudding (arroz con leche), plain 123

Rice pudding (arroz con leche), raisins 123

Ricotta cheese, part skim milk 124

Riesen® 137

Riesling 100

Ritz Cracker (Nabisco®) 128

Roast Beef Sandwich with Veggies, no mayo 156

Rob Roy 100

Rockstar Original® 111

Rockstar Original® Sugar Free 111

Rompope (eggnog with alcohol) 100

Root beer 100

Roquefort cheese 119

Rose hips 162

Rose wine, other types 100

Rum 100

Rum and cola 100

Rusty nail 100

Rutabaga, raw or blanched, marinated in oil mixture 168

Rye bread 112

Rye flour, in recipes not containing yeast 174

Rye roll 112

S

Sake 101

Salami, beer or beerwurst, beef 145

Salmon, red (sockeye), smoked 145

Sambuca 101

Sandwich cookies, vanilla 133

Sangria 101

Santa Claus melon 162

Sapodilla, fresh 162

Sauerbraten 146

Sauerkraut 169

Scallop squash 169

Scallops 146

Schnapps, all flavors 101

Schweppes® Bitter Lemon 111

Scotch and soda 101

Scrambled egg, made with bacon 142

Screwdriver 101

Sea Pak® Seasoned Shrimp, Roasted Garlic 146

Sea Pak® Shrimp Scampi in Parmesan Sauce 146

Seabreeze 101

Semolina flour 174

Sesame chicken 142

Sesame sticks 128

Shake, chocolate 151

Shake, strawberry 151

Shake, vanilla or other 151

Shallot, raw 169

Shiitake mushrooms, cooked 169

Singapore sling 101

Slim-Fast® Easy to Digest, Vanilla, ready-to-drink can 124

Sloe gin 101

Sloe gin fizz 101

Smart Balance® Light with Flax Oil Margarine, tub 119

Smart Balance® Margarine 119

Smarties® 137

Snickers® 137

Snickers®, Almond 137

Snow peas, cooked 169

Sorbet, chocolate 173

Sorbet, coconut 173

Sorbet, fruit 173

Sorghum 116

Souffle, meat 147

Soup base 142

Sour cherries, fresh 162

Sour cream 124

Sour pickles 169

Sourdough bread 112

Soursop (guanabana), fresh 163

Southern Comfort® 101

Soy bread 113

Soy chips 128

Soy Kaas Fat Free, all flavors 120

Soy milk, chocolate, sweetened with sugar, not fortified 105

Soy milk, plain or original, with artificial sweetener, ready 124

Soy milk, vanilla or other flavors, sugar, fat free, ready 124

Soybean sprouts, raw 169

Soybeans, cooked from dried 169

Spaetzle (spatzen) 149

Spaghetti squash 169

Spaghetti, with carbonara sauce 142

Spearmint tea 111

Special K® Blueberry cereal (Kellogg's®) 116

Special K® Cinnamon Pecan cereal (Kellogg's®) 116

Special K® Original cereal (Kellogg's®) 116

Special K® Red Berries cereal (Kellogg's®) 116

Spelt flour 174

Spiced ham loaf, canned 146

Spicy Italian Sandwich with Veggies, no meat 156

Spinach ravioli, with tomato sauce 142

Spinach, cooked from fresh 169

Splenda® 105

Split pea sprouts, cooked 169

Spring roll 142

Sprinkles Cookie Crisp® (General Mills®) 116

Sprite® 111

Sprite® Zero 111

Squash ravioli, with sauce 142

Starbucks® Hot Cocoa Double Chocolate 105

Starbucks® Hot Cocoa Salted Caramel, prepared 105

Starburst®, Original 138

Steak & Cheese Sandwich with Veggies 156

Stewed green peas & sofrito 143

Sticky bun 133

Stonyfield® Oikos Greek Yogurt, Blueberry 124

Stonyfield® Oikos Greek Yogurt, Caramel 124

Stonyfield® Oikos Greek Yogurt, Chocolate 124

Stonyfield® Oikos Greek Yo-gurt, Strawberry 124

Straw mushrooms, canned, drained 169

Strawberries, fresh 163

Strawberry milk, prepared 124

Strawberry pie, bottom crust only 133

Strawberry Shake 158

Streusel topping, crumb 174

Suckers®, sugar free 138

Sugar cookies, iced, store bought 133

Sugar, white granulated 138

Summer squash, cooked 169

Sunbelt Bakery® Granola Bar, Banana Harvest 116

Sunbelt Bakery® Chewy Granola Bar, Blueberry Harvest 116

Sunbelt Bakery® Chewy Granola Bar, Golden Almond 116

Sunbelt Bakery® Granola Bar, Low Fat Oatmeal Raisin 116

Sunbelt Bakery® Chewy Granola Bar, Oats & Honey 116

Sunbelt Bakery® Fudge Dipped Chewy Granola Bar, Coconut 116

Sundaes®, caramel 151

Sundaes®, chocolate fudge 151

Sundaes®, mini M & M® 151

Sundaes®, Oreo® 151

Sundaes®, strawberry 151

Sun-dried tomatoes, oil pack 169

Sunflower seeds, raw 128

Sushi, with fish 143

Sushi, with fish and vegetables in seaweed 143

Sushi, with vegetables 143

Swedish Meatballs 143

Sweet and sour chicken 143

Sweet and sour sauce 152

Sweet cherries, fresh 163

Sweet corn 152

Sweet Onion Chicken Teriyaki Sandwich with Veggies, no mayo 156

Sweet onion salad dressing 156

Sweet potato bread 133

Sweet potato, boiled 169

Sweetened condensed milk 105

Sweetened condensed milk, reduced fat 124

Swiss cheese, natural 120

Swiss cheese 120

Swiss Miss® Hot Cocoa Sensible Sweets Diet, sugar free, prepared 106

Sylvaner 101

T

Taco Bell® 7-Layer Burrito 143

Taco Bell® Beef Enchirito 157

Taco Bell® Caramel Apple Empanada 157

Taco Bell® Cheesy Fiesta Potatos 157

Taco Bell® cheesy gordita crunch 157

Taco Bell® Cinnamon Twists 157

Taco Bell® Combo Burrito 157

Taco Bell® Crunchwrap Supreme 143

Taco Bell® Double Decker Taco Supreme®, beef 157

Taco Bell® Mexican Pizza 143

Taco Bell® Nachos Supreme 143

Taco Bell® Pintos 'n Cheese 157

Taco John's® nachos 128

Taco with beans, cheese 143

Taffy 138

Tap water 111

Tempeh 169

TenderCrisp® Chicken Sandwich 151

Tequila 101

Tequila sunrise 101

Tic Tacs® 138

Tilsit cheese 120
Tiramisu 133
Toast, cinnamon and sugar, whole wheat bread 113
Toast, butter 113
Toblerone® Swiss Dark Chocolate with Honey & Almond Nougat 138
Toblerone® Swiss Milk Chocolate with Honey & Almond Nougat 138
Toblerone® Swiss White Confection with Honey & Almond Nougat 138
Toffee 138
Toffifay® 138
Tofu, raw (not silken), cooked, low fat 124
Tokaji Wine 101
Tomato juice 109
Tomato relish 143
Tomato soup mix, dry 143
Tomato, cooked from fresh 170
Tonic water 111
Tonic water, diet 111
Tootsie Pops® 138

Tortilla 128
Triple Sec 102
Triticale bread 113
Tuna Sandwich with Veggies, no mayo 156
Tuna 146
Turkey Breast & Ham Sandwich with Veggies 156
Turkey Breast Sandwich with Veggies 156
Turnip 170
Twix® 133

V
V-8® 100% A-C-E Vegetable Juice 109
Vanilla Coke® 111
Vegetable soup, condensed 143
Veggie Delite Salad 156
Veggie Delite Sandwich 156
Venison or deer, stewed 146
Veryfine Cranberry Raspberry 109
Vichyssoise 143
Vinegar 156
Vodka 102

W
Waffles, bran 133
Waffles mix 133
Walnuts 128
Watermelon, fresh 163
Wax beans 170
Weetabix® Organic Crispy 116
Wendys' 158
Werther's® Original Caramel Coffee Hard Candies 138
Wheat bran 174
Wheaties® 116
Whipped cream 106
Whipped cream, chocolate 124
Whipped cream, fat free 124
Whiskey 102
Whiskey sour 102
White flour 174
White bean stew with sofrito 143
White bread 113
White chip macadamia nut cookie 156
White chocolate Bar 138
White Russian 102
White tea 106
White whole grain wheat bread 113

White whole wheat flour 174
Whole wheat bread 113
Whopper® with cheese 151
Wild 'n Fruity Gummi Bears (Brach's®) 138
Windmill cookies 133
Wine spritzer 102
Winter melon 170
Winter type squash 170
Wise Onion Flavored Rings 128
Wrap bread 156

Y
Yams, sweet potato type 170
Yellow bell pepper, raw 170
Yellow tomato, raw 170
Yerba® Mate tea 111
Yogurt with aspartame 125
Yogurt wth sucralose 125
Yogurt, fruited, whole milk 125

Z
Zesty onion ring sauce 151
Zsweet® 138

Made in the USA
Middletown, DE
20 June 2019